SUICIDE TUESDAY

GAY MEN AND THE CRYSTAL METH SCARE

DUNCAN OSBORNE

CARROLL & GRAF PUBLISHERS

NEW YORK

SUICIDE TUESDAY
Gay Men and the Crystal Meth Scare

Carroll & Graf Publishers
An Imprint of Avalon Publishing Group Inc.
245 West 17th Street
11th Floor
New York, NY 10011

AVALON
publishing group incorporated

Copyright © 2005 by Duncan Osborne

First Carroll & Graf edition 2005

Library of Congress Cataloging-in-Publication Data is available.

ISBN-10: 0-7867-1616-9
ISBN-13: 978-0-78671-616-6

Printed in the United States of America
Interior design by Jamie McNeely
Distributed by Publishers Group West

CONTENTS

INTRODUCTION

Among gay methamphetamine users, Suicide Tuesday comes at the end of a binge. The party begins on a Thursday or Friday with the first hit of crystal. It continues through the weekend with more meth and, many users will tell you, a great deal of the best sex they have ever had, often without condoms, and, just as often, with many men.

Sleeping, eating, taking medications, either for HIV or for some other condition, may or may not be part of the weekend. By late Sunday or early Monday the user will have had enough, but that does not mean that the effects of the drug will allow him to sleep. Rest comes on Tuesday, but at a price.

A user will be physically exhausted, which is not surprising given the drug and sex marathon he has just run, but the effect is more than just extreme fatigue. Crystal stimulates the production of dopamine in the brain and it prevents the re-uptake of that "feel good" neurotransmitter as well. For the days that the user has been partying and playing, his brain has been flooded with dopamine.

The brain, just like the rest of the body, has its limits. Dopamine depletion can come at the end of a binge. That sends the user into an ugly crash that can include exhaustion and depression. It is called Suicide Tuesday because, as the name suggests, users feel so awful, they just want to die. For chronic meth users, the effect on the brain can grow making each succeeding Suicide Tuesday that much more intense and the desire to get high again that much greater.

This latest appearance of meth in the gay community has raised a great deal of concern because an unpleasant end to a binge is not the only ill effect that meth users can experience nor are meth's effects limited to those users. While these crystal using men remain a small part of the gay male community, their drug use raises a number of issues. First among these is any damage to the health of these meth users, both HIV-negative and -positive. That alone would be cause for concern.

Then meth's association with unsafe sex and the spread of HIV among gay and bisexual men is also worrisome. We know that crystal-using gay men tend to have more partners and more unsafe sex. We also know that among users the number who are already HIV-positive tends to be higher than the percentage who are HIV-positive among all gay men. The concern is that meth will fuel a resurgent HIV epidemic.

It is reasonable for the gay community to try to aid crystal users, to try to convince others to not use meth, and to try to prevent the spread of HIV among crystal users as well as among any men who may have sex with those users, but do not use crystal. What is not reasonable, in fact it is ill advised, is for the gay community to join the current hysteria over methamphetamine that has swept across America.

In newspapers, magazines, on the web, the radio, and the television, in political speeches, and meetings we are told the meth is "America's Most Dangerous Drug," that it is creating "meth babies" when pregnant women use crystal, and that it fueled the creation of new "superstrain" of HIV that now threatens gay men. These are all false.

Legal drugs, such as alcohol and tobacco, kill far more Americans every year than all the deaths associated with illegal drugs combined and cocaine, marijuana, and heroin send far more people to emergency rooms every year than meth does. There is no such thing as a "meth baby" and there is no "superstrain" of HIV.

Unfortunately, politicians, law enforcement, and the mainstream press speak much louder than those few voices that have been challenging these meth myths. These myths have taken hold in popular culture and in the minds of many Americans, including gay Americans. It is just as unfortunate that some in the gay community have joined the chorus that is promoting this mythology.

Some community leaders have said that crystal "is not a drug you can use once and put down" and meth use among gay men has been compared to the early years of the AIDS epidemic when HIV killed tens of thousands of gay men. "When gay men saw their peers' lives destroyed, it was like another HIV/AIDS plague," one advocate told the Associated Press in 2005.

The truth is far more complex than the heated words about meth suggests. Meth is a problem. In some parts of the country it is a very serious problem. This does not mean that every solution to this problem is a good one nor does it mean that every politician or bureaucrat who is talking about meth is being honest.

The meth discourse cannot be separated from America's "war on drugs." In 2014 we will mark 100 years since the

DUNCAN OSBORNE

federal government enacted the first law that was intended to regulate illegal drugs in this country. Since that time we have seen the number of illegal drugs used in this country and the number of users grow. While law enforcement has a role to play, not every action taken in the name of enforcing the law is just or right.

This current hysteria in the gay community also cannot be differentiated from the many crises that have been debated and worried over since AIDS was first noted in 1981. The gay community has a long history of seizing on an issue or a phenomenon as the cause of the spread of HIV among gay men only to let its attention lapse after a period of time. In some cases these issues were serious and, in others, they were driven by little more than sensational press coverage. One wonders if, for many gay community members, crystal is simply one more panic that will prove ephemeral.

Still, there is no question that crystal use among gay men is a problem, but those meth users have ways of using the drug and reasons for using it that will not change or succumb to a poster or a rhetorical flourish published in a magazine or a newspaper.

This is not to say that AIDS and gay groups across the country are not responding to meth use among gay men. They are and they are having success in getting men to stop using and to reduce the unsafe sex that is associated with crystal use. These groups are doing this not because of, but despite the panic that has seized the attention of some in the gay community.

There are other places in the community where people are refusing to join the meth hysteria.

My editor, Don Weise, asked me to write this book after reading an article I published in *Out* magazine in late 2004 that dealt with some of the issues I raise here. I am pleased that he did. I am grateful that Bruce Shenitz, the executive editor at *Out*, and Brendan Lemon, the magazine's editor in chief, asked me to write that story. They have continued to publish stories, as has the *Advocate*, *Out*'s sister publication, that challenge the perceived wisdom on meth use among gay men.

Much of the content in this book comes from stories I have published in *Gay City News* and its predecessor newspaper, *Lesbian and Gay New York*. I am grateful that Paul Schindler, my editor at *Gay City News*, Troy Masters, the paper's associate publisher, and John Sutter, the publisher, were committed to publishing stories about AIDS, drug use, meth and a range of related topics long before and long after other news outlets had turned to other subjects.

I am also grateful for the many people who, long before I started writing this book, were asking questions and raising doubts about drug use in America. In reading thousands of pages of Congressional testimony one of them struck me as particularly eloquent and his comments are as relevant today as they were in 1969.

When he testified before the House Select Committee on Crime, Dr. Joel Fort, a professor at the School of Social Welfare at the University of California at Berkeley, first said that "no drug is harmless, no drug is necessary for social use, and no drug is inherently desirable" then he added "There are few fields as pervaded by ignorance and hysteria as the area of mind-altering drug use and abuse. It requires no ability to claim that a drug is totally harmless or to claim that it is as dangerous as the hydrogen bomb."

I would argue that the "ignorance and hysteria" has grown louder and more pervasive since Fort testified. Our discourse, on any topic, is dominated by media companies that are often more interested in entertaining their readers and viewers that supplying them with facts and most commentators today never let what they do not know about a subject prevent them from expressing a very strong view on that subject. Given that this is the context, it should surprise no one that much of what is said or written about meth is wrong.

The gay community would do well to avoid participating in that madness. The problems that confront us, including crystal, require thoughtful and reasoned responses. Hysteria has never made any problem better.

1

AMERICA'S MOST DANGEROUS DRUG?

Sitting in the Big Cup, a coffee bar that is a popular meeting place for gay men in New York City's Chelsea neighborhood, a thirty-eight-year-old former crystal meth user described his life on the drug.

"Your sense of what seems reasonable goes out the window," he told *Gay City News* in 2004. "I was just so disgusted with my life. You keep crossing lines."

Tall and well muscled, with a light beard, he exuded an air of confidence that seemed at odds with the story he was telling. The man had smoked crystal and taken gamma-hydroxybutyrate, or GHB, a depressant, for four years. During the final fifteen months of that time, he was a daily user. He had not used either drug for fourteen months.

In the waning days of his crystal use, he found himself at a sex party for eight hours. Three other men were injecting the drug while he kept smoking.

"I was never into sex parties," he told the gay newspaper. "Then I started going to sex parties at the end . . . I went to family functions high. I volunteer somewhere. I went to that high."

The man described how on New Year's Eve of 2001 he and friends had gone to dinner. When the check arrived he found he could not perform the simple math necessary to divide the bill. A week earlier he had spent Christmas with his family and a snowstorm kept him from returning to his Manhattan apartment. He was climbing the walls as he thought about the crystal and the pipe that were waiting for him at home.

Now the man and a crew of thirty to forty recovering meth users and volunteers were preparing to engage their peers who might still be using meth. The Black Party was nine days away. The party is one of an estimated seventy-five such circuit parties that take place around the world every year and draw tens of thousands of gay men. The group planned on blanketing gay New York with anti-meth messages.

They had ten thousand palm cards and fifteen hundred posters that bore the image of a handsome young man whose face was rotting away to expose his skull. Each poster and palm card bore the text "meth = death."

They would be placed in bars, restaurants, and other businesses that cater to the partygoers. Some of the palm cards would be handed to men as they entered the Black Party. The documents listed the ill effects that can come with crystal use and information on where people who were concerned about their meth use could get assistance.

"There's a lot more to crystal than getting HIV," said the man who is HIV-positive. "It's really destructive of people's lives . . . There are a lot of negatives associated with it. We want to get across that there are a lot of dangers associated with it, but we're also trying to get across that there's a lot of help."

The group had joined a nationwide effort to combat meth use among gay men. The grisly image and the funding for their work came from the Miami-based United Foundation for AIDS, which had backed similar campaigns around the country.

"We developed a campaign called 'Meth Equals Death,'" Marc Cohen, the foundation's president, said in the same news article. "It's a very aggressive awareness campaign."

The foundation offered similar images, but with a female face or an African-American face. It had funded campaigns in Miami, Portland, Houston, Orlando, and Tampa. Groups in San Francisco and Washington, D.C., had asked to use the images.

"It has become such a serious issue in our community that we wanted to collaborate," Cohen said. "Our target audience is traveling quite a bit to different parties, different cities. The more we can do together will provide maximum exposure, provide consistent messages, and maximize the dollars that we spend."

While there had been some programs aimed at countering meth use among gay men starting as early as 1995, and largely on the West Coast, the recent efforts were notable for their visibility and reach.

In 2004 in New York City, Peter Staley, a noted AIDS activist, spent $5,000 to place anti-crystal ads with text that read "Huge Sale! Buy Crystal, Get HIV Free!" on phone booths throughout Chelsea, the heart of gay, white New York. The *New York Times* picked up the story.

Staley, who for many years was a member of the AIDS Coalition to Unleash Power, or ACT UP, was a smart activist who had always brought a special passion to his work. He had been arrested many times during ACT UP protests when he

stormed government offices or the headquarters of pharmaceutical companies. He even put a condom over the home of
Jesse Helms, the right-wing ex-U.S. Senator from North Carolina. He had also been laid low by crystal meth.

"It was a spiritual death," the forty-two-year-old told *Gay
City News* in 2004. "I was miserable. I couldn't enjoy life, I
couldn't dream about the future, I couldn't enjoy friendships,
I couldn't enjoy my relationship with my boyfriend. I was
spiritually dead."

He first tried the drug in 2000. Staley thought it was just
another party drug and he had used some of those without
side effects for many years. The meth high was remarkable
and the sex he had on crystal was extraordinary.

"It makes you feel all powerful," Staley said. "It makes you
feel young again. As soon as you're high the fact that you're
[HIV] positive just slips your mind. Any worries you have in
your life are gone. It's the perfect mid-life crisis drug because
you feel like a complete stud."

For the next two to three years Staley would return to
crystal to recapture that high and that sex. He estimated he
had thirty binges with each one lasting anywhere from fifteen
to seventy-two hours.

By the time his posters went up, Staley had not used meth
in over a year. He brought the same drive that he had applied
to his earlier AIDS activism to his anti-crystal campaign. The
purpose was to stigmatize meth and give it the "reputation it
deserves."

That was not all that the activist was doing. Staley, Dr.
Mathilde Krim, board chair of the American Foundation for
AIDS Research, a leading figure in AIDS research, and Ana
Oliveira, executive director at the Gay Men's Health Crisis,
or GMHC, one of the nation's oldest and largest AIDS

organizations, met with senior city health department officials to talk about crystal.

That meeting and the press coverage of Staley's posters prompted the health department to hastily convene a symposium in April of 2004 with New York City's health commissioner, Dr. Thomas R. Frieden, and with a group of reporters.

"The concern that we have is that, until recently, it had been much more widely used in the South, in the West, in the Midwest," Frieden said. "Over the last several years we have increasing although still anecdotal evidence that its use is increasing in New York City. The evidence is significant enough and beyond anecdotal in some cases that it tells us it is a significant potential problem here."

In a matter of months, the city also produced $300,000 to fund anti-meth ads at three local AIDS groups.

One of those groups, HIV Forum, was established in July of 2003 by Dan Carlson and Dr. Bruce Kellerhouse. The two gay men were friends who had been talking about unsafe sex among their peers. Carlson, the younger of the two, reported that the men he met often insisted on having sex without condoms.

"I would say 'I'm becoming very disillusioned, another person wanted to have unsafe sex with me,'" Carlson said in 2003. "I talked about my own personal experience in meeting a lot of people who wanted to have unsafe sex with me and becoming, at times, rather persistent about that."

Kellerhouse, a psychologist in private practice, was concerned about what his friend was telling him and he was seeing his clients becoming infected with HIV.

"We were having dinners and lunches and spending time together and a lot of it was being spent complaining about the lack of HIV prevention messages," he said. "Initially it became around what Dan's experience was and over the most recent months it had become less so. It became more focused on what is the community doing for us, what is the city, what are the organizations, all of the structure that has done prevention, what are they doing for us?"

By the spring of 2005, the men had produced eight town meetings in New York City. Three were concerned with crystal though the drug was discussed at every single meeting.

They drew their largest crowd in late 2004 when Larry Kramer, the playwright and longtime AIDS activist, spoke at Cooper Union. Their second largest crowd, perhaps as many as eight hundred people, turned out for "The Crystal Meth-HIV Connection," the second meeting they produced in early 2004. In that audience were staff from the federal Centers for Disease Control and Prevention, or CDC, and activists from as far away as Florida and Massachusetts.

The Crystal Meth Working Group, a part of the HIV Forum, eventually produced its own poster campaigns in 2004. The first one, "Crystal Meth: Nothing to Be Proud Of," contrasted pride celebrations in 1994, which marked the twenty-fifth anniversary of the Stonewall riots, and those celebrations in 2004, which were represented by the image of a young man smoking meth, sitting in front of a computer, and, presumably, searching for sex partners.

The ad was placed throughout some of New York City's gay enclaves—the West Village, the East Village, Chelsea, Hell's Kitchen, Harlem, and Williamsburg—and it ran in the *Advocate*, a national gay magazine; *Next*, a New York City glossy; and the Gay Day Disney Guide.

The working group loaded a larger version on the back of a billboard truck and marched with it down Fifth Avenue during New York City's 2004 Gay Pride March.

"It is meant to shock," Carlson said in a 2004 press statement. "We want to shatter the complacency and break the silence around HIV infection and crystal meth. We have to learn to take care of each other as a community because nobody else is going to do it for us. Things don't have to be like this."

A second series of posters from the working group featured hot, shirtless young men posed and looking into the camera. The text declared them to be "Crystal Free and Sexy." These ads were placed on phone booths up and down Manhattan's Eighth Avenue, Chelsea's main drag, and published in gay press outlets.

The working group soon began receiving calls from AIDS groups and local health departments around the country who wanted to use their ads for anti-meth efforts. In late 2005, Carlson said that meth had taken over his group's work.

"Crystal has co-opted our health agenda," he said in the September issue of *Out*, a national gay magazine.

Before the HIV Forum had begun its work, AIDS and gay groups across the country held town meetings on meth and the numbers of meetings only grew in 2004 as the gay community became increasingly aware of the crystal meth problem.

Crystal meth moved GMHC to establish a task force in early 2004 to study the drug. Among the seventeen task force members were Richard Burns, executive director of the Lesbian, Gay, Bisexual, and Transgender Community Center, Dennis deLeon, president of the Latino Commission on AIDS, and other leading figures in New York City's AIDS and gay communities. Many had fought for lesbian and gay rights for decades.

When the task force issued its report after sixty days,

among its recommendations was a call to the community to "articulate and promote the view that defining and limiting unhealthy behavior is not tantamount to placing limits on gay sexuality or placing limits on gay identity and freedom."

In a community that long prized its sexual freedom, that charge was a radical departure from the view that preserving gay men's sexuality is a paramount value. Concern about meth had moved leading members of New York City's gay and AIDS communities to describe the behavior of some gay men as "unhealthy" and they suggested that limits on that behavior could be appropriate though they likely avoided any controversy by not saying what those limits might be.

"That's actually a pretty out-there statement for traditional AIDS activists to sign on to and I was pleased to see it," said Staley, one of the task force members, in *Gay City News*.

The gay and lesbian community actions came at a time when America's war on drugs was increasingly targeting methamphetamine. All of the weapons that had been aimed at other drugs, such as heroin, crack, and marijuana, were being applied to crystal. However inadvertently and with the best of intentions, the gay community had joined the anti-meth chorus.

In 1999, members in the U.S. House of Representatives established the bipartisan Congressional Caucus to Fight and Control Methamphetamine and by 2005 it had grown to 103 members. The caucus members took their message to the National Press Club, to conventions and meetings, and to the press across America.

In a 2001 issue of *Reason* magazine, Mark Souder, a Republican Congressman from Indiana who chairs the House Subcommittee on Criminal Justice, Drug Policy, and Human Resources and a caucus member, called meth "a monumental problem for America." The demands for a government response by the members of the Congressional meth caucus were almost always accompanied by a request for more cash for their districts.

The caucus members tended to represent Western and Midwestern districts, often rural or suburban areas, that had recently experienced the types of drug-related crime, including violent crime, that was typically associated with drugs in American cities. The caucus members, the communities they represented, and law enforcement in those communities blamed meth.

Not only did they have to deal with crime, local law enforcement also had to contend with cleaning up the small home labs that users constructed to supply themselves with crystal. In this case, meth was represented as an environmental problem because of the waste that was generated and haphazardly discarded by these lab operators.

In July of 2005, the National Association of Counties released two surveys, one of local law enforcement and a second of child welfare agencies, and declared that "Sixty Percent of Counties Report Meth as Largest Drug Problem" in a press statement. The responding agencies were largely rural and suburban counties.

The media also weighed in. The press represented users as neglecting themselves and their families. Their homes were usually filthy and sometimes littered with pornography that they used while high. They suffered from "meth mouth," a condition supposedly resulting from poor dental hygiene during crystal binges. They were difficult to treat with a high rate of recidivism.

The big gun for the anti-meth crusaders—meth babies— emerged in 2000. These stories took the "crack baby" template that was created in the 1980s and simply substituted meth for crack cocaine.

In some of these stories, the children were living in homes where meth was used or manufactured. In others, the children were born to mothers who had used meth while they were pregnant. In all these stories, the phenomenon was presented as threatening the children and placing a burden on state and local agencies that protect children.

What may be the first story on this subject was distributed by the Web site www.apbnews.com in 2000 under the headline, "Meth Infants Called the New 'Crack Babies.'" It reported on the "increasing number of methamphetamine-addicted babies in area hospitals" in Des Moines, Iowa. In 2001, the *Chicago Tribune* published "Methamphetamine Rise Sparks Worry for Babies."

Some stories bordered on the absurd. In 2004, the *Minneapolis Star Tribune* quoted a social worker asserting that when pregnant women use meth their "babies can be born with missing and misplaced body parts" and "she heard of a meth baby born with an arm growing out of the neck and another who was missing a femur." These and similar stories continued into 2005.

The corollaries to the "meth baby" story in the gay community were persistent rumors of crystal-fueled gang rapes at parties during which the victim inevitably was infected with HIV and increased aggression during domestic violence incidents in same-sex households.

As is the case with all such tales, they had a grain of truth. Children are threatened by meth, crime and meth do exist together, there is rape and domestic violence among gay men, but whether these things are related or even exist to the degree portrayed by politicians or the press remains a question.

Sometimes these stories are used for reasons that are not apparent, such as defending government budgets. This was illustrated in 2004 when two reporters[1] from *Gay City News* met with Anthony P. Placido, special agent in charge of the federal Drug Enforcement Administration's, or DEA, New York Field Division.

Placido began by noting that he had just ended a conference call with the DEA's administrator during which they had discussed a cut to the agency's meth enforcement budget that had been proposed by the Bush administration. That was a concern, Placido noted, because meth labs in homes were adversely affecting the children who lived in those homes.

This was an odd assertion given that no meth labs had been found in New York City, where the newspaper is distributed, nor was this likely to be a concern for most of the gay community. That these were DEA talking points became apparent four days later when the *New York Times* published a story titled "Home Drug-Making Laboratories Expose Children to Toxic Fallout" on its front page.

Generating this sort of press coverage is a standard gambit in budget and policy battles though news consumers are rarely informed of such motivations in these stories. The DEA was not doing anything that other bureaucracies and politicians had done before. Notwithstanding any such motives, no one can reasonably deny that meth is a problem, but the extent to which government's response to meth, or any issue, is driven by bureaucratic needs or the degree to which press coverage increasingly tries to be entertaining cannot be dismissed as an influence in the meth discourse. That discourse hit a high note in 2005.

The Bush administration had been battered for several years over its response to meth with much of that criticism

1. Paul Schindler, my editor at *Gay City News*, and I attended this meeting.

coming from fellow Republicans. In August of 2005, the White House sent John Walters, director of National Drug Control Policy, Attorney General Alberto R. Gonzales, and Michael Leavitt, the secretary of the U.S. Department of Health and Human Services, to a drug conference to defend its meth policies and introduce a new meth initiative. Souder, who has held repeated hearings on crystal dating back to 1998, dismissed the effort.

"We're looking for a scream, not a peep," he said. "This proposal, unfortunately, doesn't have anything new in it. At my last hearing they waived a report with a list of recommendations, and this was all in it."

The next day, the DEA announced it had arrested 164 people in three countries and four American cities who were part of an extensive drug smuggling operation. The press release announcing the arrests, titled "DEA Fractures Major Meth Pipeline into U.S.," noted that the group moved "four thousand pounds of cocaine, twenty to thirty pounds of heroin, and in excess of fifty pounds of methamphetamine on a monthly basis throughout the United States."

This was primarily a cocaine smuggling operation, but the political pressure being brought to bear on the White House required a different spin. The mainstream press dutifully reported that the DEA had smashed a meth smuggling ring.

If the anti-meth chorus reached a crescendo in 2005, the opponents also grew louder that year. In August of 2005, *Newsweek* published a cover story on meth that declared that the drug was "America's Most Dangerous Drug." Commentators and media critics from both the right and the left assailed the piece as hyperbole and wrong on some facts.

John Tierney, the conservative *New York Times* columnist, offered a general critique of the "meth epidemic" in a column several days after the *Newsweek* piece appeared. Referring to the "law-enforcement officials and politicians who lead the war against drugs," Tierney wrote, "Like addicts desperate for a high, they've declared meth the new crack, which was once called the new heroin (that title now belongs to OxyContin). With the help of the press, they're once again frightening the public with tales of a drug so seductive it instantly turns masses of upstanding citizens into addicts who ruin their health, their lives, and their families."

That same month, a group of leading researchers "with many years of experience studying prenatal exposure to psychoactive substances, and as medical researchers, treatment providers, and specialists with many years of experience studying addictions and addiction treatment" published an open letter objecting to the "meth baby" coverage.

The authors asserted that there was no science to support the view that "meth babies" were real and they pointed out that there was long experience showing that "crack babies" were not. After "twenty years of research" there was no "recognizable condition, syndrome, or disorder that should be termed 'crack baby'" nor had studies on crack use by pregnant women "found the degree of harm reported in the media and then used to justify numerous punitive legislative proposals." They also disputed claims that meth was hard to treat and that users experienced a high rate of recidivism.

"Similarly, claims that methamphetamine users are virtually untreatable with small recovery rates lack foundation in medical research," they wrote. "Analysis of dropout, retention in treatment, and reincarceration rates and other measures of outcome, in several recent studies indicate that methamphetamine users respond in an equivalent manner as individuals admitted for other drug abuse problems."

The gay community was not immune to the hysteria surrounding meth. The overheated rhetoric that is used when raising the alarm over a health issue was applied to crystal. Crystal use was an "epidemic" or a "growing threat" to gay men.

In 2005, the book *Tweakers: How Crystal Meth Is Ravaging Gay America* told the stories of "more than 250 crystal users and those who treat them." As the title suggests, these were gruesome stories that described lives that no one would envy and no one would want to live. Whether they represent "gay America" is another question.

By 2005, it had become routine in speeches, books, and media reports to describe crystal and its impact on the gay community in only the most negative terms and to suggest that that impact was being felt community wide. There was certainly no shortage of people who were willing to offer those views.

Joe Camper, the director of VALEO, a treatment center for lesbians and gay men at Chicago's Lakeshore Hospital, told the *Chicago Tribune*, "This is a drug you cannot use recreationally. When they say 'meth equals death,' they're not kidding. Every aspect of your being is virtually destroyed by this drug. I don't think I can say that in strong enough terms."

Sophie Godley, prevention director at Boston's AIDS Action Committee said in the *Boston Globe*, "So many of us know people whose lives have been destroyed by crystal meth, people whose lives have just crumbled in a short period of time."

Cleve Jones, the executive director of LA Shanti, an AIDS service organization in Los Angeles, told the *Los Angeles Times*, "Our community is being destroyed."

Jones is a heroic figure in the gay community. He survived the early years of the AIDS epidemic and was among those who built the infrastructure of nonprofit groups that today

serves people with AIDS in California. His experience in the
AIDS epidemic made his comment to the *Times* all the more
poignant.

"For ten years I lost loved ones, every week in the papers,
there were three pages of obituaries," he said. "I survived all
this, and now we're continuing to be destroyed by this
drug."

That rhetoric and the anti-crystal actions were being challenged by some in the community. The May 2004 issue of
Genre, a national gay magazine, featured a news analysis piece
that, while not dismissing crystal's harm, suggested that some
recent responses to the drug were more sensational than based
on facts.

In the fall of 2004, *Out* published a story[2] that noted that
many illicit drugs used by gay men were harmful and associated with unsafe sex and pointed out that the population of
gay men who used meth tended to be poly-drug users. Taking
their meth away would not stop their risky sex, the piece
asserted. Another *Out* story, this one published in 2005, also
raised doubts about the focus on meth.

After his posters appeared in 2004, Staley found himself in
a debate with proponents of harm reduction, a philosophy
that argues that a drug user need not quit using to lessen a
drug's damage, who argued that his efforts at demonizing
crystal were effectively demonizing crystal users. When he
spoke at the HIV Forum's town meeting on crystal, some of
those harm reduction advocates challenged him on this point.

Donald Grove, a senior staffer at New York City's Harm
Reduction Coalition, said the message would ultimately be,
"There is a group of people out there, the ones who continue

2. I authored this story.

to use, who don't matter . . . Let's be real about the role that demonization and stigmatization play."

Even some of the community activists, such as Carlson and Staley, who had produced their own poster campaigns, challenged some anti-meth efforts.

In late 2004, David N. Kelley, the U.S. attorney for the Southern District of New York, announced that his office would produce its own anti-crystal posters. Using pictures of convicted dealers and text that included their six- or seven-year prison sentences, the posters asked, "Was it worth it?" They were to be displayed "in areas where the individuals did their drug dealing, including the Chelsea neighborhood where many of the drug deals took place," according to a press statement.

The community activists saw that their posters were about to be associated with a law enforcement campaign that would surely anger many in the community and they made a quick, and successful, lobbying effort to have Kelley abandon his plans for the posters.

"People were just furious," Staley said. "They looked like wanted posters of gay men."

A 2004 town meeting, organized by the HIV Forum, on crystal and law enforcement revealed a similar sentiment. The panel featured a senior DEA special agent, a defense attorney, a harm reduction advocate, and federal and state prosecutors. The law enforcement agencies received a chilly reception.

"I would like to see the gay community say, 'No, we will solve our own problem,'" said one audience member during the event, which was held at New York City's gay community center. "We don't need you."

Toward the end of the evening the state prosecutor asked, incredulously, "There are predators who are targeting your community and you are telling us that you don't need us?" That drew calls of "That's right" from the audience.

There was some community resistance to meth hysteria, but what was lacking in much of the discussion on meth was an accurate description of the extent of the problem. Horror stories and an excessive reliance on law enforcement sources had replaced facts though these were readily available.

Data from the federal Substance Abuse and Mental Health Services Administration, or SAMHSA, reported that 1.9 million Americans sought drug treatment services in 2002. Over 800,000 people reported a problem with alcohol or alcohol and a second drug. Just under a quarter million had a cocaine problem; marijuana was the problem for 290,000; heroin for 289,000; and 126,000 were battling amphetamines. That national data, however, disguises the meth problem.

Citing the SAMHSA data in a 2005 online column, the Portland *Oregonian*, which had produced a series on meth in 2004, reported that in 2003, "seventeen states treated more people for methamphetamine abuse than for cocaine or heroin." Those states were predominantly in the West. Meth was a growing problem.

"In the remaining thirty-four states and Washington, D.C., treatment admissions rose by an average of 200 percent from 1999 to 2003," the newspaper reported. "The total number of people in treatment for meth nationally almost doubled during the period, from 73,000 to 136,000. By comparison, the number of cocaine treatment cases rose by 2 percent, to 251,000."

There was similar growth in other statistics. The federal Drug Abuse Warning Network reported that in 2000 meth was mentioned during emergency room visits 13,505 times. That number climbed to 17,696 in 2002. While that is a significant increase—31 percent—the number is still well below the 199,198 emergency room mentions of cocaine in 2002, the 119,472 mentions of marijuana, and the 93,519 mentions of heroin.

During that same period of time, the mentions of cocaine increased by 14 percent, mentions of marijuana increased 24 percent, and mentions of heroin fell by about 1 percent. The DAWN and SAMHSA numbers include all users of those drugs and not just gay and bisexual men.

Then the harm of all illicit drugs pales in comparison to those that are legal. The best estimates are that alcohol kills 85,000 Americans every year and tobacco kills 435,000. Nicotine is still America's most dangerous drug.

While meth use among gay men is undeniably a serious problem, the extent of its use by those men remains unclear and, where there is data, it varies widely from city to city. Some data shows one number when gay men are asked about any use and a much smaller number when they are asked about recent use, a pattern that is similar to that found among all Americans.

The same *Globe* story that quoted Godley cited a 2004 study of one thousand gay men by the Massachusetts health department that found that 10 percent reported using meth at least once in the prior year and 2 percent said they used the drug once a week.

The *Columbia Chronicle*, a student newspaper of Columbia College in Chicago, cited a 2001 study that put meth use among gay men there at 7 percent with 2 percent reporting monthly use. More recent data, cited by David McKirnan, a researcher at Howard Brown Health Center, a gay health clinic in Chicago, in the same story reported that 18 percent of five hundred HIV-positive men interviewed by the clinic in 2004 had used crystal.

In 2004, the health department in Seattle began a "comprehensive review of local behavioral research studies" and included in that an effort to measure crystal use among gay and bisexual men there. The department found that roughly 10 percent of those men had used meth in the past year with use of the drug being two times higher among men under thirty and three times higher among men who were HIV-positive. Roughly 2 percent of the meth users had injected the drug in the past year and 11 percent of the current users in the study were injectors.

In 2003, the Associated Press described a California study of 63,098 gay and bisexual men that found that 10.5 percent, or 6,637 of the men, had used crystal. That number could be artificially low because it measured men throughout the state. The rate in San Francisco or Los Angeles, just two California cities with large gay male populations, is probably higher. A 2003 article in the *San Francisco Chronicle* said health officials there estimated that up to 40 percent of gay men in that city had tried crystal.

Studies in New York City done by the Center for HIV/AIDS Educational Studies and Training at Hunter College and the Center for Health, Identity, Behavior, and Prevention Studies at New York University found that anywhere from 6.8 percent to 22 percent of the study participants reported recent meth use.

Between 1990 and 1997, meth use among gay and bisexual men in American cities from the West Coast to the East Coast was estimated to range from 5 percent to 25 percent, according to a 2000 study by the Hunter College center that was published in the *Journal of Homosexuality*.

Just as the prevalence of meth use among gay and bisexual men varies from state to state and city to city, it likely varies among the different populations of those men who live in those cities.

The Seattle health department reported that in 2004 "methamphetamine use is more prevalent among white [men who have sex with men] than [men who have sex with men] of color," which suggests that in Seattle, meth is favored by white, gay men. The popular perception is that it is a white, gay man's drug and studies support that though, clearly, African-American, Latino, and Asian gay men use the drug.

A 1999 study done by the NYU center and published in 2000 looked at forty-nine gay and bisexual New York City men who used crystal. The sample was not random, but a convenience sample—meaning the men were actively recruited because they possessed certain attributes, such as a particular race or ethnicity. Just under 45 percent of the men were African-American, Latino, Asian, or of mixed race or heritage.

In 1999, there was little discussion of meth use in New York City and certainly little awareness that the drug was being used, but the study authors found their participants in just forty-eight days, which suggested that meth was already popular among men of all colors. They also learned that the African-American men had to travel to Chelsea, a largely white, gay enclave, to buy their crystal and that white, gay men "used significantly more crystal in comparison to African-Americans."

Other evidence suggests that gay meth users are a diverse population. At a 2005 town meeting about meth held at the National Black Theater in Harlem, Dr. L. Jeannine Bookhardt-Murray, the medical director at Harlem United, an AIDS service organization, told the crowd, "This drug has made its way across the country and uptown."

The meeting included testimony from Michael Kelly, an

African-American man, a meth user, and, a "harm reduc-
tionist" who said he used the drug successfully.

"Certain drugs can be used intelligently and without the
bad effects the doctor described before," he said, referring to
Bookhardt-Murray. "If you use it, please use it intelligently."

In 2005, the Latino Commission on AIDS released a report
that found meth users in its client population. The LCOA
clients used the drug or wanted to use it because that would
get them into the Chelsea gay scene.

"From our focus groups, it seems that for many immigrants
it's a rite of passage," deLeon said. "It's a way to become part
of the New York City Chelsea gay community. Because drug
use is so much a part of the culture the feeling is that to
become part of the New York gay community crystal meth is
part of that."

Testifying before the New York City City Council in 2004,
a member of Crystal Meth Anonymous said that the recovery
group needed "to start our first Spanish-language meeting
since a growing number of our members are native Spanish
speakers."

The CMA member said that the group was searching for
space outside of a gay community organization because, as
more heterosexuals came to CMA meetings, the group
needed space that would be completely comfortable for these
new members.

In 2005, speaking at a day-long conference in New York
City sponsored by Housing Works, an AIDS service group, a
different CMA member told the crowd that the group's membership in New York City was made up of gay men, lesbians,
and straight women.

At the same conference, Dr. Perry N. Halkitis, a psychology professor at New York University and a co-director

at the NYU center, described the state of meth use in New York City.

"It is a drug that crosses racial lines, ethnic lines, HIV status," he said.

In the studies of gay and bisexual male meth users, the men have ranged in age from their teens or younger to their fifties and older. Their meth use varied from occasional to frequent. Their use was associated with sex, safe and unsafe, and sometimes not. They were swallowing it, injecting it, smoking it, putting it up their asses in gel caps like suppositories, or removing the needle from a syringe and injecting meth mixed with water up there, a practice called booty bumping. Often they were doing other drugs, sometimes many other drugs, when they were doing crystal.

One thing is clear from all these studies and data. They strongly suggest that most gay and bisexual men are not using methamphetamine. Just as the threat posed by meth can often be exaggerated, these studies present evidence that a segment of the gay male community is in serious trouble with the drug and very much in need of the wider community's help.

The growth in CMA meetings in the gay community demonstrates that. A quick look at the organization's online meeting schedule showed that in most large American cities there is at least one CMA meeting that is listed as a gay and lesbian meeting or meets at an institution that traditionally serves the lesbian and gay community.

As one reads the schedule, starting with Hawaii and moving toward the East Coast, that trend becomes even more pronounced until one hits Philadelphia, Atlanta, Miami, New York City, or Boston where the CMA meetings are almost entirely associated with gay community institutions.

There are many reasons to be concerned about the meth

use among gay and bisexual men not the least of which is the impact of the drug on these users.

Unlike drugs such as marijuana or peyote, which are plants that are dried, then smoked or eaten, methamphetamine cannot be said to be natural. Crystal is the result of a chemical manufacturing process. While the manufacture, possession, and sale of the drug are illegal, the meth manufacturing process is effectively unregulated. There is no equivalent of the Food and Drug Administration ensuring that meth has a certain purity and is free of contaminants. While dealers likely have no desire to poison or kill their customers, when purchasing meth, the controlling principle must be buyer beware.

The most commonly used methods of manufacturing crystal are the anhydrous ammonia method and the red phosphorus hydriodic acid method, according to DEA information. Both methods use ephedrine or pseudoephedrine, a drug that is widely used in over the counter cold remedies, as a chemical precursor. As the names suggest, the processes use some noxious chemicals and can include household items such as aluminum foil, battery acid, Drano®, and matchsticks.

A 1991 study by Gary Irvine, an environmental health supervisor at the Seattle health department, and Dr. Ling Chin, an epidemiologist at the National Institute on Drug Abuse, or NIDA, included a long list of chemicals that are "associated with illicit methamphetamine manufacture" that reads like the contents of a toxic waste dump. The DEA estimates that for every pound of meth produced in a lab, five to ten pounds of chemical waste are left over. A number of mainstream press reports examined the proliferation of this waste across the country caused by manufacturers simply dumping it by a roadside. A meth user might be exposed to these chemicals when he or she gets high.

A 1991 study by Dr. Brent T. Burton, the medical director at the Oregon Poison Center, noted fourteen cases of lead poisoning that resulted from crystal use. Burton could not say if the cases were caused by a chemist doing an occasional bad job or if lead was consistently present in the drug, but even at low levels, the fourteen users consumed so much meth that the lead levels in their bodies reached a point where it made them sick.

"It is unknown if lead poisoning from methamphetamine is episodic, due to poor technique, or is more widespread, but at a lower level of toxicity," he wrote.

These chemicals are not simply dangerous because they can make users and manufacturers ill. Some are volatile. The DEA reported that in 2002, 694 clandestine meth labs across America exploded or burned down. During his 2004 testimony before the City Council in New York City, the DEA's Placido noted that just days before, a hotel in Indiana was evacuated after a meth lab in one room burst into flames.

The purity of meth can also vary tremendously. The DEA reported that between 1994 and 2001, the average purity of seized meth samples dropped from just under 72 percent to just over 40 percent. More recently, the agency reported that meth purity levels in California samples ranged from 10 percent to 100 percent in 2004. In Seattle, the DEA reported that average meth purity had climbed from 30 percent in 2001 and 2002 to 50 percent in 2004 with some samples in that final year getting as high as 66 percent. A user cannot be certain as to the quality of the product he or she has purchased.

Part of the problem may be that, while the DEA estimates that 80 percent of the crystal used in the United States is manufactured in so called "super labs" that can generate ten pounds or more of higher purity crystal in a twenty-four-hour production cycle, there remain large numbers of small labs that are manufacturing the drug.

In 2003, the DEA shut down 142 super labs, which are usually associated with Mexican organized crime groups, and more than ten thousand so called small toxic labs. The small toxic labs produce smaller quantities, often for local sale, and can be run by people who are also meth users. They also tend to be inexperienced manufacturers.

The problems associated with meth use are not limited to the environmental consequences and potential exposure to toxic chemicals. A number of studies have documented a range of health problems that can result from meth use. These include strokes, heart attacks, seizures, and irregularities in one's heartbeat. Meth can induce psychosis, depression, and paranoia. The drug does cause overdoses and it has killed users.

There are other seemingly minor health effects that former users will say were actually significant. Some health experts have noted the tendency of meth users, actually users of any sort of uppers, to grind their teeth. This can lead to long-term dental problems, including the loss of those teeth.

Some speed users, including those who use crystal, experience "formication," or the hallucination that insects are crawling beneath their skin. They then pick at their skin to get at the imagined bugs, creating sores that are called "speed bumps" or "crank bugs." This can cause abscesses, infections, and scarring.

These health concerns are not the sole possible consequences that a user may face. One is the presumed connection of crystal with crime and violence. The view that meth users are more prone to violence and criminal behavior dates back decades though there is no data to support it other than anecdotal evidence.

The meth-violence connection came to the fore in the lesbian and gay community with a unique angle—the occurrence of gang rape among gay and bisexual male meth users—and a more standard one, the link between domestic violence and crystal.

Gang rape among gay meth users was for some time a rumor that one would hear. Typically, the story was of a user whose life had been ruined by meth and had gone on what would be his last binge where he was assaulted and infected with HIV. Former users would occasionally report having heard of it. These stories were inevitably second- or thirdhand, but in a 2005 article in *Gay City News*, the first cases were reported.

Sam Orlando, vital service care coordinator at New York City's Lower East Side Harm Reduction Center, told the newspaper that he was aware of two gang rape cases that involved crystal. One victim was a friend of his and the second was a center client.

"He was with a couple of people," Orlando said of the client. "They did some crystal. They went to a party. They did some more crystal. He said he was raped. I don't know by how many guys."

The same article cited staff at New York City's Gay and Lesbian Anti-Violence Project noting an increase in domestic violence that is associated with meth.

"We are seeing more domestic violence that is related to methamphetamine," said Victoria Cruz, a coordinator of domestic violence and sexual assaults at the agency. "There is an increase related to methamphetamine."

Staff there were seeing not just more domestic violence cases, which involve crystal, but the perpetrators who were using the drug tended to be more violent.

Jeannette Kossuth, a rape and sexual assault counselor

there, said, "What we're seeing is an increase in the nature of the violence. It's becoming more violent."

Generally, law enforcement and social service agencies across the country have reported that meth is associated with violent crimes, domestic violence, and child abuse or neglect. That may only be a perception, it may only be rhetoric or it may be that users who commit crimes would have done so whether they used crystal or not. No data establishes the relationship.

"There is a belief that methamphetamine is more associated with violence, particularly with domestic violence and child abuse," said Dr. Richard A. Rawson, associate director of the Integrated Substance Abuse Programs at the University of California Los Angeles. "As far as I know there have not been any data yet to confirm that . . . We've looked at the criminal justice data to see if we can find any evidence of meth users perpetrating more violent crimes, but we haven't found it."

As law enforcement increasingly turns its attention toward meth, gay men have been arrested, prosecuted, and imprisoned. In February 2004, Kelley announced the indictments of eight men who had been selling meth and other drugs in the gay community.

"We're not here to just announce an arrest or filing of charges as we typically do so much as we are here to discuss a new challenge for law enforcement as well as the community at large, particularly the gay community," the federal prosecutor said at a press conference.

By the summer of 2005, all eight had pleaded guilty. Some had been sentenced others had been jailed pending their sentencing hearings. They were facing serious prison time. If fifty grams of pure crystal or five hundred grams of mixed product can be tied to a person, he or she can face a mandatory sentence.

"Under the statute, if you have this amount or if this amount can be attributed to you there is a ten-year mandatory minimum," Isabelle A. Kirshner, a criminal defense attorney, said in 2004.

The mandatory minimum federal sentence for selling five grams is five years. A dealer need not sell those amounts at one time. Those minimums can apply when one person has sold a total of fifty or five grams over an extended period of time. Federal judges have very limited discretion in applying these sentences. For instance, if the crime was not violent or did not involve a gun, some time can be taken off the mandatory minimum sentence.

Kirshner had represented a number of gay men who had been arrested for dealing crystal and she raised the alarm about the potential results of an arrest for dealing meth.

"I'm seeing a lot of young, gay men who are getting arrested for crystal meth who appear to be completely ignorant about the incredibly serious consequences," she said. "The bottom line is that a lot of these guys are very sympathetic, they don't have criminal records, but there is not a lot that judges can do."

At his press conference, Kelley reported that federal law enforcement in New York City made eleven meth arrests in 2002, but "in the last six months alone we have made . . . thirty arrests involving over twenty-five pounds of the drug with a street value in excess of over $2.5 million dollars."

The DEA also entered the fray in 2004. In that interview with *Gay City News*, Placido said that the crystal problem in New York, while serious, was relatively small in comparison to the trafficking in heroin or cocaine. The DEA had investigated the eight men in an effort dubbed "Operation Chelsea Connection."

When Placido spoke at the Kelley press conference, just six days after his interview with the gay newspaper, he reiterated the view the crystal was not a major problem in New York City, though he promised more cases.

"This is the beginning rather than the end of our efforts in this area," he said. "Fortunately the abuse of methamphetamine, which has reached epidemic proportions in some parts of the country, has not reached those levels here in New York. We hope there is still time to really stem the tide."

When he testified before New York City's City Council, just two months later, Placido's view had shifted.

"I can tell you that our investigation revealed that the abuse of this drug in the gay community may be much more prevalent than we had previously imagined," he said. "We are currently investigating at least ten separate organizations that are distributing methamphetamine within the five boroughs of New York City."

Many of the investigations "share common characteristics" in that the groups were moving "multiple kilogram loads" of meth into New York City from other parts of the country and they are importing other drugs as well.

"My office has obtained evidence and received intelligence which indicates that methamphetamine is becoming more widely available in New York's club scene," Placido said. "We are increasingly concerned that methamphetamine will join the ranks of ecstasy or MDMA, [GHB], and ketamine as widely abused party drugs."

Local law enforcement in New York City also reported more meth cases. In 2003, the state Office of Special Narcotics, which prosecutes drug felonies throughout the city, prosecuted just three cases. By mid-2004, it had eight cases.

Elsewhere around the country, the picture was similar. In May of 2005, Richard M. Daley, Chicago's mayor, announced that the city would launch an anti-crystal effort.

"Methamphetamine is both a public health problem and a law enforcement problem," Daley said in a press statement. "It's important that we raise awareness of its dangers, reduce its use on the North Side and keep it from spreading across the city."

Police would conduct "more undercover operations to identify the sources of the drug," train "police officers to recognize signs of methamphetamine manufacture and use," and educate "club and tavern owners on how to identify users and keep the drug out of their establishments."

While Daley said that meth "is not confined to the gay community," the city noted that its strategy included "leaders of the lesbian, gay, bisexual, transgender community."

In 2004, at the United Foundation for AIDS, Cohen established the South Florida Crystal Meth Task Force to "track the drug's usage and manufacture in the region," the *Miami Herald* reported. The task force included "several health and law enforcement officers."

While gay men have been using methamphetamine for decades, it appears that federal and state law enforcement agencies have only recently begun to investigate meth sales in the gay community. That may be due, in part, to the dealers being non-violent and keeping a relatively low profile.

In a 2004 *Gay City News* article, Bryant Seifried, fifty-four, said that in the 1980s and 1990s, he was one of five dealers who were supplying most of the crystal to the gay community in southern California. They knew each other and there were no fights among them.

"There were no guns, there was no violence, there were no territories," said Seifried, who is gay. "We were acquaintances . . . None of us were arrested, none of us felt threatened. The labs were getting busted."

Seifried's dealing began in the 1980s when he was supplying friends with small amounts of the drug.

"I was helping my friends out," he said in an interview in the Coxsackie Correctional Facility, a maximum-security state prison in New York. "It just grew. It became this monster until I was making fifty thousand a month. I did very well."

Eventually, he was dealing in pounds of the drug and, "from the late 1980s all the way up through the 1990s," selling meth was his primary source of income. In 2001, he was prosecuted for sending shipments of meth to a network of seven New York dealers in an investigation run by the DEA and the Office of Special Narcotics.

Seifried received a sentence of four years to life. Four of the New York dealers—John Polcari, forty; Christian Sandy, thirty-two; Robert Stone, thirty-nine; and Ray Wasyl, forty-seven— were given shorter prison sentences. Two of the remaining three defendants were given five years probation and one was placed on probation for life.

It is apparent from the indictment in the case—dubbed the "Transcontinental Mail Order Crystal Meth Corporation" — that the network had been thoroughly penetrated by police. An undercover police officer or officers made repeated purchases of large amounts of meth from the dealers starting in August of 2000 and ending in February of 2001. Their phone calls were either observed by police or tapped.

The indictments in Operation Chelsea Connection, the arrests announced by Kelley, paint a similar picture. The indictment for six of the defendants noted that on January 27,

2003, a co-conspirator, who was not named in the case, traveled from California to New York City to deliver six pounds of meth to Jeffrey D. Watson, forty-two, a Chelsea resident. The agency knew that Watson kept the drugs in a storage locker in the basement of his apartment building.

The cash deposits made by Watson, John R. Warner, forty-one, and Joseph J. Burns, thirty-one, between March and November of 2003 at three different banks, and totaling more than $410,000, were listed in the indictment. The men were charged with trying to avoid federal bank reporting requirements by keeping their deposits to small amounts.

The DEA knew the dates and details of phone conversations and in person talks the men had among themselves and with their three fellow dealers, Avon Chandler, thirty-four; Gregory C. Smith, forty-two; and Angel Garcia, thirty-eight. The agency detailed the amounts of meth the men sold, when and where those sales took place, and the dollar amounts paid for those drugs.

The other two Operation Chelsea Connection defendants—James Urinyi, thirty-four; and Gary Kiss, forty-three—were arrested after a "confidential informant," listed as "CI–1" in the indictments, assisted the DEA in making purchases both from the two men and, in conjunction with Kiss, from a dealer in Atlanta during June and July of 2003.

"CI–1," who was later identified as Peter K. Harris, forty-three, had pleaded guilty to "various narcotics offenses, is currently awaiting sentencing, and is providing information to law enforcement in order to receive consideration on his/her criminal case," according to the indictments. The DEA had hidden a video camera in Harris's apartment and taped the transactions. Harris was arrested after he sold meth to a confidential informant identified only as "John" in court records.

Becoming an informant may be the only way to avoid the harsh federal sentences.

"Cooperation is the cornerstone of the federal system," said Kirshner, the criminal defense attorney, at the forum on crystal and the law. "It's the only way to get around mandatory sentences."

The Harris case illustrated just how irrational such deals can be. All three men were meth users. Urinyi, like Harris, had agreed to become a confidential informant, but he began using meth again, which violated his deal. In such cooperation deals, the defendant pleads guilty to the top count against them and if they violate the deal, they are sentenced under that top count. Urinyi was given 121 months, or just over ten years, in November of 2004.

Harris stayed clean, completed his cooperation agreement and, in July of 2005, walked out of court a free man after serving just a few months in prison. He had to forfeit $167,000 he made from selling meth plus another $13,000 in cash that was found in a safe in his home and a safe deposit he kept in a bank. He was given four years on probation.

Kiss refused to cooperate, but he did stop using and he enjoyed strong community support. A large number of former crystal users and friends wrote to his judge and appeared at his sentencing. He was sentenced to five years in federal prison, five years of supervised release when he completes his prison sentence, and a $70,000 fine in June of 2005.

The cases involving two Harris co-conspirators had the same feature. The sentences appeared to have as much to do with the crime as whether the defendant produced valuable information for the federal government or stayed clean.

In 2004, Ronald "Sammy" Watkins, thirty-five, was sentenced to eighty-seven months in prison, or just over seven years, and five years probation after he sold meth to John on three occasions in early 2003.

Watkins was diagnosed with bipolar disorder, or manic depression, in 1992 and had been under the care of a psychiatrist and a therapist during that time though he often did not take his prescribed medications, according to court records. Like many people with mental illness, Watkins used other drugs. He used meth, cocaine, crack, alcohol, and Special K for years and had tried, with limited success, to end his drug use. Watkins was diagnosed as HIV-positive in 1994 and by the time of his sentencing in 2004 he had progressed to an AIDS diagnosis.

Watkins's attorney argued that his bipolar disorder and his health should lead to a reduced sentence, but Jed S. Rakoff, the federal judge in the case, rejected that argument.

Another co-conspirator, Kurt Douglas Guiterrez, thirty-five, was sentenced to 121 months, or just over ten years, and five years of supervised release though Guiterrez, a native of Belize, will likely be deported when his prison time is up. He brokered meth sales.

"I was the contact person involved in the sale of methamphetamines between the buyer, John, and the seller, Watkins and Harris," he said at a June 2003 hearing. Guiterrez was also a meth user.

"In the mid-1990s, he entered into drug use that ultimately turned into drug addiction," Rakoff said of Guiterrez at his 2003 sentencing hearing.

Hans Reynoso, twenty-nine, was identified as one of Watkins's drug suppliers and was sentenced to time served and three years of supervised probation after he entered into a cooperation agreement with the government.

Judging by these and other cases, small informal networks

and individual dealers appear to be typical of meth sales in the gay community. Many of these dealers are gay and meth users themselves.

The cases demonstrate that the time in which men could deal drugs in the gay community and believe that they are simply helping gay men party, perhaps even party safely, are clearly gone. Unlike the dealers who dominate the cocaine, heroin, and marijuana markets, the dealers in the gay community appear to be no match for the federal, state, and local law enforcement officers who have long practiced their skills against serious and committed drug dealers.

"Law enforcement is crashing the party that has gone on virtually unnoticed by them for years," Carlson said in 2004. "There are now potentially life-changing legal consequences to openly expressing a desire to use crystal meth."

There is one bright spot in this bleak picture. While drug sentences in the states can be just as severe as the federal terms, every state now has a drug court program that diverts low-level users into treatment and away from prison, according to the National Conference of State Legislatures.

"The principle behind drug courts is they give judges discretion," said J. Blake Harrison, a policy specialist at the conference. "If [the offenders] complete their treatment, they can get their charges dismissed or reduced."

As of September 2004, there are 1,212 drug courts operating in the U.S. with 476 drug court programs being planned, according to the National Criminal Justice Reference Service, a program of the U.S. Department of Justice. Some of those state drug courts are funded by the federal government. A few states, such as California and Arizona, mandate that low-level drug offenders be referred to treatment, according to Harrison.

Meth users can face these physical and legal. They may find themselves homeless or unemployed. They may see relationships with friends, family, and partners end as those people become fed up with the user's behavior or the user may find the drug to be more important than loved ones and friends and abandon those people.

With some exceptions, all of these consequences can be reversed or ameliorated. Prison sentences will end. Relationships can be repaired. People who are homeless and unemployed can be hired and housed. There are some effects of crystal use that are or may be irreversible—the drug's effect on the brain and HIV infection.

One of the most serious health effects, and certainly one of the most widely discussed, is crystal's impact on the brain. That effect may be central to why some use meth in the first place.

At the Housing Works conference, Dr. Antonio E. Urbina from New York City's St. Vincent's Hospital and Medical Center described meth's effect on the brain. Crystal causes the release of dopamine in the brain and inhibits dopamine re-uptake, giving users a double dose of that "feel good" neuro-transmitter, according to Urbina.

"You get a huge surge of dopamine," he said.

Some users, particularly those who may be dealing with depression or other serious mental illness, may use the drug because, among other reasons, they crave that dopamine surge to alleviate the unpleasant feelings they are experiencing.

In studies in rats, mice, nonhuman primates, and people, however, crystal has been shown to deplete or damage those parts of the brain that produce dopamine. The depression that follows the meth use can be that much worse because the user has damaged that part of the brain that could contribute to his or her feeling better. This might explain what is often cited as the very high recidivism rate among meth users.

The user is trapped in a cycle of euphoria when high, where he is engaged with sex partners in a desirable social setting, followed by a crushing depression that he seeks to fix with more meth, which is followed by another depressed episode, and so on.

This is a simplistic rendering of what is a complicated process in the brain. It could be that meth is only partly responsible for the damage to the brain and that other related processes cause harm as well. One thing is certain—depression and meth are linked.

Chronic use can lead to "major depression," Urbina said. In one study, 62 percent of the meth users remained depressed two to five years after they stopped using the drug, according to Urbina.

"You are going to damage your brain and it may be something you don't get back," Urbina said.

Several studies that have used positron emission tomography, or PET scans, to map the brains of meth users have produced disturbing results. PET scans create a picture of a certain molecular activity in the brain.

The PET scans of the meth users, admittedly a small number, showed large black spaces where parts of their brains were not functioning. In some of these studies, the subjects were people who had used large amounts of meth for an extended period of time. Some of the users had consumed an incredible one to two grams daily for years.

A 2004 study from the NIDA noted that some users reported experiencing a "lack of motivation and anhedonia" for up to two years after they stopped taking meth. "Anhedonia" is exhibiting a lack of pleasure in an activity that had once been pleasurable. The same study noted that some, but only some, of these effects could be reversed. But it is HIV and crystal that are of greatest concern among researchers and doctors, and within the gay community.

For men who are already infected with HIV, crystal may have a harmful effect on their immune system, though it remains unclear if that results from some as yet unknown action of the drug or if it results from users failing to adhere to the rigorous dosing schedules of anti-HIV drugs when they are high. When HIV-infected individuals miss doses, the virus can develop resistance to those drugs, which can increase the individual's viral load, a measure of the amount of virus in their blood.

That is not a small thing. There are just twenty drugs currently available to treat HIV. Many of those drugs have noxious side effects that render them intolerable to some people with HIV. A crystal user who misses enough doses of enough drugs and develops a resistant virus could find himself with far fewer choices for treatment of his HIV.

Gay men who are HIV-positive and using crystal are potentially subject to all of the unpleasant consequences that the drug can create and then those men may face one that is unique to them.

Some data suggests that meth and some proteins in HIV are toxic to the neurons in the brain that release and take up dopamine. That could mean that a meth user, particularly one who is not taking anti-HIV drugs, is facing a two-pronged attack on that part of the brain, one by crystal and the other by the virus.

A 2002 study of feline cells that were infected with a virus that was similar to HIV and then exposed to meth found a fifteen-fold increase in the ability of that virus to replicate and mutate. Those findings have not been replicated in human beings, but the implications are that meth could play a role in HIV's assault on the brain and HIV-related dementia.

Some HIV-negative, sexually active gay and bisexual men who use meth and cruise Web sites, bathhouses, bars, sex clubs, and other places for sex partners have to be concerned with HIV. A 2005 study from the NYU center definitively linked crystal use to new HIV infections in some of the study participants.

"Many studies have documented associations between meth use and sexual risk behavior," Halkitis said. "In this particular study, we have a bunch of men who have seroconverted and we were able to link their seroconversion to their sexual behavior to their meth use."

The study looked at the club drug use of 450 gay and bisexual men in 2001 and 2002. Sixty-five percent of these men, or 293, reported recent meth use. Among the 293 men, 101 were HIV-positive. The other 192 said they were HIV-negative or they did not know their status, but ten of these men tested positive for the virus. The ten men were called "seroconverts" in the study.

The seroconverts reported eighteen days of meth use in the four months before participating in the study while the other 182 meth users reported only twelve days of use. The real difference between the seroconverts and the other meth users was in reports of unprotected, receptive anal sex, the type of sex that is most likely to transmit HIV.

When the seroconverts were not high on crystal, they had only a little more unprotected, receptive anal sex than the other meth users, but when they were high on crystal, the seroconverts reported an average of 18.78 of these sex acts

while the HIV-negative men averaged 1.64 acts of unprotected, receptive anal sex when high.

"When they are high it goes through the roof," Kelly A
Green, a co-author on the study said. The meth-using seroconverts are likely using the drug to ease feelings of loneliness'
or depression.

"The implication is that these may be men who are so
dependent on this drug to be with other men that when they
are with those men they lose all inhibitions," Halkitis said.
"That feeling of isolation and depression are absolutely key."

Another study, called EXPLORE, of 4,295 gay and bisexual
men in six American cities produced a similar result though
not the definitive link that Halkitis found. The study, which
ran from 1999 to 2001, found that 2.1 percent of the men
were infected by the end of that time, the *New York Times*
reported in February 2005.

While a number of things accounted for those new infections, including unprotected sex with many partners or
injecting drugs, the men in the study who used meth were
twice as likely as those who did not use the drug to become
HIV-positive.

"This was a really surprising finding," Dr. Grant Colfax, a
principal investigator on the study and a director in San Francisco's Department of Public Health, told the *Times*. "There's
reason to think there's a combination of factors involved."

A 2002 survey of 786 gay and bisexual men in New York
City, conducted by Hunter College center, reported that the
crystal users were 3.5 times more likely to report unprotected
anal sex with a partner of a different HIV status in the ninety
days before taking the survey than men who did not use
crystal.

Studies dating back to 1987, through the 1990s, and into

the twenty-first century have also found that meth, unsafe sex, and possible HIV infection are linked. Generally, the gay and bisexual men who use meth are more likely to report more partners, more unprotected sex with those partners, and just more sex than men who do not use the drug. All of this—the drug's toxicity, its connection to HIV—explains why meth has been vilified in the gay community.

What is very clear is that meth is a serious problem in the gay community. It can harm the users in a variety of ways and some of the ill effects may be permanent. It is just as clear that America is in the grip of yet another panic over a drug and that some in the gay community are joining that hysteria.

This current panic, however, is concerned with a drug that has been used by Americans, including gay men, for decades and while there have been concerns expressed about speed in the past it has never before received the sort of attention it is garnering today.

Uppers have never had an esteemed place in popular culture, but they were certainly embraced. The drugs were viewed by doctors and pharmacists as useful in treating a range of disorders. Meth, as a demon, is a relatively recent phenomenon.

2

SPEED: THE DRUG
WE ONCE LOVED

"Maybe you've heard about Benzedrine," an anonymous musician wrote in "On a Bender with Benzedrine" in the September 1946 issue of *Everybody's Digest*, a popular magazine. "Most writers on the subject have blandly concluded that the tricky stuff is safely guarded from misuse. But I, and a few thousand others in the entertainment field, know differently."

The musician had been introduced to Benzedrine one night by a colleague named Hal, a pseudonym, when "five of us sagged at a table near the bandstand" and "all of us were wondering what we could do to pep up a bit." Hal had the answer. "Ever tried a benny?" he asked his friends. At the next break from playing, one of the five was sent to a nearby drugstore to buy a fifty-cent Benzedrine Inhaler. The product had been introduced to American consumers by Smith, Kline & French Laboratories in 1932.

The inhalers were also marketed to doctors in publications such as the *Journal of the American Medical Association* where physicians were told that "Benzedrine Inhaler therapy does not spread infection." The inhaler was a vapor while liquids "may carry pathogenic organisms from affected to uninvolved tissues," the doctors were warned in one 1947 ad.

The inhaler was supposed to be used to treat the symptoms caused by allergies and colds, but many consumers had taken to using it for a different effect. The musician and his friends tore open the inhaler, pulled out the Benzedrine-laced paper inside, and dipped the paper into their beer for about fifteen seconds.

"Better take half a strip, first time," Hal warned them. Twenty minutes later the men were high. "I'll take my next chorus while floating around the ballroom," the musician quoted one saying. Another said, "Brother, I'm as light and strong as twice myself."

The group stayed up all night talking, though "the subject didn't matter; each of us babbled away happily." When they stopped by a local diner for their usual after-performance meal they found that they were not hungry. This was a source of great amusement as they noted that one of them, Red, had a waistline that was "bulgy and bennies would carve him down."

Benzedrine was just one of what would become, by 1971, roughly four hundred types of speed being sold in the United States In 1946, the musician noted that Benzedrine was being used by students when cramming for an exam, truck drivers on long trips, and the U.S. military to keep soldiers and pilots awake. He wrote that there had been "a few deaths, perhaps, from Benzedrine intoxication," but generally, his ominous opening lines notwithstanding, the musician had little to report about Benzedrine that was negative. When he spoke with a colleague from "big time entertainment circles," he learned that the drug was very popular.

"Bennies are old stuff to show people I've met all over the country and in all branches of entertainment," the colleague said. "Their hours of work and their temperament are largely responsible, I suppose. Some of the best-known performers wouldn't be without Benzedrine, and, of course, a few go overboard."

It was not just entertainers who were using Benzedrine. Three years after the Benzedrine Inhaler was introduced, "sales rose to over fifty million units" per year, wrote Carol A. Spotts and James V. Spotts in *Use and Abuse of Amphetamine and Its Substitutes*, a 1980 book.

The practice of opening the inhaler and using the paper inside was common. The musician wrote that when he and his friends opened their Benzedrine Inhaler, the manufacturer had printed a warning in blue ink on the paper inside telling consumers that the drug was for "inhalation only, not for internal use, and is dangerous when swallowed."

Only someone who ripped open the inhaler would see the warning. Clearly, Smith, Kline & French Laboratories knew how some Americans were using their product. The company was not the sole distributor of such inhalers.

In a 1947 article in the *Journal of the American Medical Association*, Dr. Russell R. Monroe and Dr. Hyman J. Drell wrote that while amphetamine in pill form was available only by prescription, users had found and were availing themselves of the over-the-counter inhalers. That year, there were at least four on the market. All of them could be taken apart and the drug could be obtained from the cotton or paper inside. Users would chew these, swallow them, soak them in coffee, water, or an alcoholic beverage and drink it, or tear the paper into little pieces and mix it with chewing gum. It was a highly effective method of getting cheap speed.

Monroe and Drell had a volunteer dip the inside of an inhaler in coffee for just ten minutes and then drink the coffee without swallowing the paper. Amphetamine was detected in his urine just under two hours later and it was still detectable five days later.

These drugs, however, were not vilified in the press or popular culture. On the contrary, they were celebrated. Monroe and Drell wrote that a jewelry manufacturer sold a charm bracelet with an attached pillbox in U.S. newspapers, using the tagline, "For Benzedrine if you're having fun and going on forever; aspirin if it's all a headache."

In 1944, Harry "The Hipster" Gibson recorded "Who Put the Benzedrine in Mrs. Murphy's Ovaltine?" a song that the *New York Daily News* called a "showstopper" in a brief 2004 biography of Gibson. The song never answered the question, but Benzedrine gave Mrs. Murphy a new lease on life. There also appeared to be a great deal of doping going on in the Murphy household. The same song asked, "Who put the Nembutol in Mr. Murphy's overalls?"

The use of uppers likely extends back centuries to the time when the first South American chewed a coca leaf or an African did the same with khat. The Chinese have brewed tea from ma huang, the source of the ephedrine used in U.S. pharmaceutical products in the early twentieth century, for thousands of years. The Ethiopians are credited with discovering coffee. These cultures have legends and folk tales associated with these substances, which suggest that their use, either for medicinal purposes or simply for pleasure, is well established and accepted.

The first manmade, amphetamine-like substances were reported by a chemist in Germany in 1887, according to *The Amphetamines: Their Actions and Uses*, a 1958 book by

Chauncey D. Leake, a professor of pharmacology at Ohio State University. A Japanese chemist, identified only as A. Ogata in studies, synthesized methamphetamine in 1919 and Burroughs Wellcome received FDA approval to sell injectable and pill forms of the drug, under the trade name Methedrine, in the United States in 1944.

There appears to have been little activity related to these drugs for the first two decades of the twentieth century. A single study in 1910 noted the effect that stimulants had on blood pressure, but it was not until the 1920s that interest in them became apparent.

In 1924, Dr. Ko-Kuei Chen, a pharmacologist at the University of Wisconsin, described that action of ephedrine on the body and two years later the *New York Times* reported that Chen had developed a new way of isolating ephedrine from ma huang. Chen's drug would be a "powerful aid in the hands of modern physicians" in treating colds, hay fever, as an anesthetic, and for raising blood pressure, the university announced. The race to produce synthetic ephedrine had begun.

In 1926, Eli Lilly and Company, which eventually had its own inhaler on the consumer market, made its first ever graduate fellowship award to Robert H. Herbst, a chemist. The *New York Times* reported, "He will conduct research on the development of synthetic methods for preparing alkaloids of the ephedrine type."

For the pharmaceutical industry, producing synthetic ephedrine was a priority. There was a significant U.S. market in drugs to relieve colds and hay fever, but the supply of ma huang from China was inconsistent, a problem that grew more pronounced in 1937 when Japan invaded China. The supply problems were serious enough then to prompt comment from the U.S. Department of Commerce, which noted that the 90,000 pounds of ma huang shipped to the United States in July of that year would likely be the last shipment for some time.

The following year, the commerce department disclosed that "three German firms" had manufactured synthetic ephedrine. In 1939, researchers at Purdue University announced that they had made synthetic ephedrine.

Ephedrine was not the only upper that was of interest to the pharmaceutical industry. In 1927, Gordon A. Alles, a chemist, working with George Piness, a Los Angeles allergy specialist, synthesized the first amphetamines. According to Leake, "Alles assigned his patents to the Smith, Kline & French Laboratories" in order "to advance the clinical use of the drug." The company gave the drug the trademark name Benzedrine though that name, or bennies, its shorter version, later came to refer, in popular usage, to any type of speed.

The pursuit of speed was not an academic exercise. The market for these products, and for drugs in general, was only growing larger and, much to the frustration of the pharmaceutical industry, a great deal of the money spent on drugs of any type was not being paid to the established pharmaceutical manufacturers.

In 1932, the year the Benzedrine Inhaler was introduced, Dr. Robert P. Fischelis, president of the New York chapter of the American Pharmaceutical Association, told a gathering of his colleagues that Americans were spending $715 million a year on drugs with much of that cash being "spent unwisely and often dangerously," the *New York Times* reported.

One hundred and ninety million dollars annually went for prescription drugs, $165 million went for home remedies, and $360 million was spent each year on "patent medicines," Fischelis said.

Press reports throughout the 1930s and 1940s document the highly competitive nature of this market and show the pharmaceutical industry releasing new products, usually containing ephedrine, during that time. Today, the market for these over-the-counter cold and allergy products is estimated to be between $1 billion and $3 billion a year. Most of these products still contain ephedrine or pseudoephedrine.

Colds and hay fever were not the only disorders and conditions that were being treated with amphetamines. While they were not presented as wonder drugs, they were close to that in the view of some medical professionals. In a 1937 lecture at the New York Academy of Medicine, Dr. William Healy, the director of a "guidance center" in Boston, suggested that Benzedrine could act like high-octane gasoline and move the human brain to achieve greater things. "The extraordinary energy-stimulating powers of Benzedrine sulfate . . . appear to prove that the potential of the brain cells is far from being fully realized under ordinary conditions of nutrition or stimulation by what the bloodstream has to offer," Healy was quoted by the *New York Times*. "When Professor Edgar Douglas, Nobel prize winner, of Cambridge University, speaks of the new world we might live in if our brains were twice the present size, one is led to think of what we might achieve if only through feeding our cerebral tissues with better hormonic and other activating materials we could realize the full working powers of what we already have."

At a time when drug testing was largely unregulated, researchers and doctors began treating a great variety of conditions with uppers. Their use was explored throughout the 1930s to the 1970s. Possible applications included treating opiate addiction or overdose, alcoholism, narcolepsy, epilepsy, spastic colon, seasickness, Parkinson's disease, senility, post-operative recovery, obesity in adults and children, or to alleviate some of the unpleasant effects of pregnancy. Psychiatry also considered amphetamines as a treatment for depression, psychosis, or schizophrenia.

In 1936, Dr. Abraham Myerson, a psychiatrist who worked at the Massachusetts State Hospital, announced that Benzedrine had a "very remarkable influence" on people contemplating suicide. The American Medical Association gave its stamp of approval to Benzedrine for the treatment of narcolepsy and "postencephalitic parkinsonism" in 1937, the year that speed in pill form first came on to the U.S. market.

In 1938, Dr. Wilfred Bloomberg, a neurologist at Boston City Hospital and an instructor at Harvard University, declared that Benzedrine was a cure for alcoholism. The next year, however, the Associated Press quoted Bloomberg warning wives against "slipping a tablet of the compound into their husband's coffee" to cure their drinking. "We can't assume that Benzedrine or any single thing is a cure for alcoholism, but tests have shown that the compound provides an interval of sobriety which allows doctor and patient to establish a sound relationship for more fundamental treatment," Bloomberg said.

The calming effects of amphetamines on hyperactive children were noted in the scientific literature as early as 1937 and that use was explored for decades. In 1940, the *New York Times* reported that Dr. Charles Bradley and Margaret Bowen presented data at a meeting of the American Orthopsychiatric Association on one hundred "problem children," seventy-seven boys and twenty-three girls, ages five to twelve, who had been treated with Benzedrine. "The behavior of fifty-four of the experimental children became 'subdued,'" the *Times* reported. "Dr. Bradley and Miss Bowen think that the drug acts by imparting such a sense of well-being that conflicts are no longer irritating." Using uppers on "problem children" did not stop there. A 1937 study and another in 1952 investigated the effectiveness of amphetamines in treating bedwetting in children. The treatment involved dosing the child subjects just before bedtime.

By 1946, one study in "Use and Abuse of Amphetamine and Its Substitutes" listed thirty-nine clinical uses for amphetamines, including schizophrenia, alcoholism, depression, "morphine and codeine addiction," "night blindness," "caffeine mania," and "restless legs."

By 1971, there were 102 known drugs that contained only amphetamine or methamphetamine and another 291 drugs that contained either of those drugs in combination with others. There were 393 brand-name drugs available to U.S. consumers and doctors manufactured by 204 companies, according to *Use and Abuse of Amphetamine and Its Substitutes.* In 1969, Fred A. Coe, Jr., president of Burroughs Wellcome, told the House Select Committee on Crime that methamphetamine is sold "alone and in combination with other drugs by over seventy companies."

Americans were certainly using those drugs and had been for years. Testifying before the Senate Subcommittee on Narcotics in 1955, Thomas Jefferson Scott, a commodity specialist at the U.S. Tariff Commission, reported that U.S. pharmaceutical manufacturers produced 52,000 pounds of amphetamine base in 1953. That was enough base to produce roughly 4.7 billion five-milligram doses. In 1949, the industry produced enough base for 1.4 billion doses.

In 1962, an FDA survey of the drug industry estimated that 4.5 billion ten-milligram amphetamine doses were produced annually in America and half of them were diverted to users who did not have a prescription. Two major amphetamine manufacturers, Parke-Davis and Eli Lilly & Company, were not included in that survey.

Five years later, 12 million U.S. adults, roughly 6 to 8 percent of the population, were getting uppers by prescription, according to a study cited by Dr. Jonathan O. Cole of the Massachusetts Department of Mental Health at a 1970 conference on amphetamines held at Duke University. There were 23.3 million prescriptions for uppers filled that year—10.8 million were new and 12.5 million were refills. Eighty percent of the amphetamine prescriptions written in 1967 went to women. "Rarely have drugs with so few medical indications been so widely prescribed," Cole wrote.

Dr. Everett H. Ellinwood, from Duke's School of Medicine and a conference organizer, agreed. "Medically prescribed amphetamines comprise 14 percent of all psychoactive drugs sold by prescription in this country, a percentage that is far out of proportion to the specific and valuable use of these drugs," Ellinwood wrote. Amphetamine use was so widespread in the 1960s that Ellinwood cautioned that a patient who presented as a "paranoid schizophrenic" in a hospital emergency room would have to be examined for amphetamine use given that the drug's symptoms could resemble that disorder.

Another estimate, cited by Marisa A. Miller, a director at the National Institute of Allergy and Infectious Diseases, a unit of the U.S. Department of Health and Human Services, in an article in *The American Drug Scene*, a 2004 book, put the legal American production of amphetamines at 3.5 billion pills in 1958 and climbing to ten billion pills by 1970. There were 31 million amphetamine prescriptions written in 1967, according to Miller. While the Cole and Miller estimates disagree, one thing is certain. By 1967, tens of millions of Americans were using legal speed.

By the 1950s and 1960s, the federal and state governments were just beginning to regulate the legal drug marketplace. There were few brakes on the desire for uppers, but this consumption of speed was not driven solely by great demand, a supply to match it, and loose or no federal and state laws. However inadvertently, the U.S. government participated in creating the market for these drugs when it gave uppers to its troops during World War II and later conflicts.

Miller cited an estimate that during World War II roughly 200 million amphetamine pills were given to American troops. Both the U.S. and British military studied the use of uppers on troops during the 1940s, 1950s, and 1960s. These drugs were used to keep soldiers alert or to prevent seasickness in sailors. Most of the warring nations during World War II used uppers to aid their troops.

"All of the important combatant nations in World War II used these drugs judiciously in aviation, especially during prolonged and hazardous bombing missions." wrote Dr. Maurice H. Seevers, a pharmacology professor at the University of Michigan Medical School, in *Amphetamine Abuse*, a 1968 book. At the time, the use of speed by the U.S. military was unremarkable.

In an article published in the *New York Times Magazine* in 1945, First Lieutenant Wilfred N. Lind, a B–29 pilot, described the experience of flying missions in the Pacific. He wrote that while he and his co-pilot had the luxury of turning on the plane's autopilot and taking a nap, his navigator could not rest and needed a boost to stay awake. "The automatic pilot is great help to everyone, but the navigator," Lind wrote. "He just rubs his tired eyes, takes some more Benzedrine, and goes to work again."

The anonymous musician, who published in *Everybody's Digest* in 1946, noted that U.S. troops had used speed and cited the consequences of that use in the lives of discharged soldiers. "Deathly-tired combat troops have taken 'power pills' for that extra effort which clinched a bitterly won position," the musician wrote and added later, "It has been suggested that discharged war veterans who failed to find jobs, had strained relations with loved ones, or felt inadequate to adjusting to social life would search out Benzedrine to bolster flagging energies and dispel apathy. Veterans are using the stuff, all right. I've seen this first hand in a social club where I was playing in the orchestra."

Monroe and Drell, in their 1947 study, interviewed 1,081 inmates at an Indiana military prison and found that 264, or 24 percent, admitted to amphetamine use. Among the users, 89 percent had started using in the previous four years, which suggests that their use began during their military service. Just under 39 percent of the users indicated they planned on continuing to use amphetamine when they were released.

During the Korean War, which raged from 1950 to 1953, American troops were issued uppers and they encountered methamphetamine when they took leave in Japan.

During World War II, Japan's pharmaceutical industry had produced millions of doses of the drug which were used by the military and civilians who were supporting the military in manufacturing and other similar industries. When Japan surrendered in 1945, those drug companies simply dumped their remaining product on the market. "After the war, the contract for a large amount of methamphetamine which had been stored by pharmaceutical companies for military use was canceled," according to one study in *Use and Abuse of Amphetamine and Its Substitutes* by a Japanese researcher. "The companies tried to sell these stocks on the open market by advertising the drug as one that would inspire the fighting spirits in daily life."

Roughly two million Japanese, out of a population of 89 million, were involved with meth by 1954. The Japanese government enacted new laws in 1948 and 1951 that were intended to crack down on the drug with the result that illegal meth labs began operating. Additional laws were enacted in 1954 and 1955. By 1957, meth cases in Japan had been dramatically reduced. "Two unfortunate consequences resulted from our use of amphetamines during World War II," wrote John William Rawlin, a sociology professor at Southern Illinois University, in *Amphetamine Abuse*. "First of all, we helped to create a serious problem in Japan through careless disposal of drugs there; and second, our own problem was aggravated when ex-servicemen who had been introduced to amphetamines during the war brought their knowledge home to civilian life."

The military's use of speed continued well into the 1960s. In a 1970 report from the House Select Committee on Crime, the Pentagon reported that it had purchased just under eighty-two million ten-milligram doses of amphetamine in 1966.

The army bought just under 23.6 million doses, or 19.6 pills for each member of the army, the navy bought 33.5 million doses, or 33.3 pills for each sailor, and the air force purchased just under 24.5 million doses, or 27.5 pills for each member of the air force. By 1969, the defense department had reduced its purchases of uppers to just under 32 million doses. Some air force pilots used speed as recently as 1991 during the Gulf War.

Given that millions of Americans were using speed it is no surprise that gay men and lesbians were also using these drugs. In 1955, U.S. Senator Price Daniel of Texas, chair of the Subcommittee on Narcotics of the Committee on the Judiciary, held a series of hearings across the country on "Illicit Narcotics Traffic," as the hearings were titled.

In Los Angeles, Louis P. Walter, a captain in that city's police department, told the subcommittee that gay men and lesbians had a particular taste for speed and that was a concern. "I would like to make an observation that I feel is accurate, in my opinion," Walter said. "I have found in connection with our arrests for amphetamines and that type of stimulant drug that to a great extent the homosexual males and females both have an affinity for that type of thing. It is not confined, of course, exclusively to them, but it does seem to have an incidence greater amongst those people in that connection, and in connection with the fact that we do find it used by teenagers there is a concern in that regard, that this amphetamine seems to be used by adult people of degenerative characteristics, immoral people."

That same year, Congressman Hale Boggs of Louisiana, chair of the Subcommittee on Narcotics of the House Ways and Means Committee, held his own series of hearings and heard similar testimony from Kenneth E. Monfore, chief of the FDA's Seattle district office. That office and the Seattle police had learned of a local drugstore that was selling amphetamines illegally. They arrested four men who had been selling the drug on disorderly conduct charges. "We were advised that the four arrested were known to the police as confirmed homosexuals," Monfore said. "The arrested men admitted that they had been obtaining amphetamine sulfate through one of the drugstores in the skid road section of the city."

Monfore and the local police then conducted an undercover operation in a local bar to determine the extent of drug sales there and to find the sellers. "Through the cooperation of the police department and one of the men arrested, our inspectors dressed themselves in the type of clothing common to that of the homosexual crowd and frequented the skid road tavern where, according to the information obtained, these drugs were being promiscuously distributed following their purchase in larger quantities from the suspected drugstore," Monfore said.

It was "the leaders of those who frequented the tavern hangout" who were selling the drugs, but, Monfore assured the subcommittee, no young people had been given the drug. "Although our investigation did not directly disclose that these dangerous drugs were being sold or distributed to juveniles, our inspectors did observe that juveniles were hanging around outside of the tavern in question and on occasion the juveniles left the area accompanied by one of the known homosexuals," Monfore said.

A number of studies in *Use and Abuse of Amphetamine and Its Substitutes*, dating from 1961 to 1976, reported on gay men and lesbians who were using speed. A 1961 study, titled "Amphetamine Addiction and Disturbed Sexuality," had a sample of fourteen patients, eight men, aged twenty-nine to forty-nine, and six women, aged twenty-two to thirty-eight. The authors wrote that "overt perverse sexuality including homosexuality was present in 29 percent of the cases prior to addiction . . . In 36 percent of the cases, sexual drive was markedly increased while using amphetamines . . . Some addicts used amphetamines for this very purpose and were thereby enabled to perform extraordinary feats."

A 1969 study in England of seventy-four regular meth injectors, 80 percent were male and 20 percent were female, found that half of the women and 19 percent of the men "admitted to homosexuality." Then in New York City, in 1970, a study reported on three homosexual men, aged twenty-eight to thirty-two, who used Wyamine, an inhaler product similar to the Benzedrine Inhaler, and were admitted to Bellevue Hospital suffering from psychosis. All three men had learned how to use the Wyamine inhaler from friends.

One man had been admitted to Bellevue eight times in the prior months with "Wyamine-related paranoia" the cause of seven of those admissions. The drug made him feel he was being pursued and he would attract the attention of the police to aid him. A second had been admitted to Bellevue sixteen times in the prior twenty-three months. He was diagnosed with "acute drug psychosis" and "chronic schizophrenia." When high, he would stand on street corners and deliver sermons. The third man had five Bellevue admissions in the prior two-and-a-half years.

A 1976 study on the "Clinical Effects of Amphetamine and L-DOPA on Sexuality and Aggression" had a sample of sixty New York City patients, included forty-three men, aged eighteen to thirty-seven. Of the men, eleven, or 26 percent, were "practicing homosexuals at the time of hospital admission," and some of the forty-three men resembled current meth users. "Eight males reported 'marathon' sexual relations resulting from a combination of intensified sexual feelings and delayed ejaculation," the authors wrote.

Other evidence is merely suggestive of gay and lesbian community involvement with amphetamines. In his 1969 study of speed use and violence in the Haight-Ashbury section of San Francisco, Dr. Roger C. Smith, from the University of California at San Francisco, wrote that while heroin addicts constituted "the bulk of speed users in the late 1950s," other groups began to use the drug, including "others on the criminal or bohemian fringe of the Tenderloin and North Beach areas of San Francisco."

In the 1950s, the Tenderloin was San Francisco's gay ghetto. Presenting at the 1970 Duke conference, Ellinwood asserted that the use of illegal speed in San Francisco had sprung up in some of the less expensive hotels in the Tenderloin. "The 'far out' activities, sexual and otherwise, of the addicts who congregated in these hotels provided the basis for the term 'speed freak,'" Ellinwood wrote.

Similarly, Greenwich Village, the New York City's gay center during the 1950s and into the 1990s, was presented in *Amphetamine Abuse* as the locus of speed use in the city in a study by Seymour Fiddle, a sociologist affiliated with the East Harlem Protestant Parish. "I gather from my interviews that the Village is an area of greatest concentration of both amphetamine and amphetamine abusers," Fiddle wrote. He also interviewed a young meth user, identified only as John, who told Fiddle that he could no longer buy the drug uptown. "[T]hese neighborhoods around mine where the kids use 'em—they're dry—nobody can get 'em," John said. "Everybody's goin' down to Greenwich Village—that's where they get 'em."

Certainly some of the gay or bisexual men who were part of Smith's "bohemian fringe" were known to use uppers. The poet Allen Ginsberg wrote "Kaddish," an elegy for his mother, in 1958 while under the influence of methamphetamine, according to *Dharma Lion: A Critical Biography of Allen Ginsberg*, by Michael Schumacher.

Ginsberg was with a friend, Zev Putterman, in mid-November of that year, when he was introduced to meth. "He had chippied some morphine and methamphetamine, the latter a new experience for him, and he was feeling both energetic and nostalgic as the night edged toward the early hours of the morning," Schumacher wrote. Ginsberg left Putterman's Manhattan apartment at dawn and returned home. He began writing the poem, pausing only to eat and take Dexedrine tablets "when he felt his energy flagging." The poem was written in a single session that stretched from 6:00 A.M. on a Saturday until 10:00 P.M. the following Sunday. According to Schumacher, "In all, he filled fifty-eight pages, many marked by tears that fell onto the paper as he wrote."

John Wieners, also a poet and a contemporary of Ginsberg, was living in San Francisco in 1958 when he wrote "A Poem for Benzedrine" and *The Journal of John Wieners Is to Be Called 707 Scott Street for Billie Holiday, 1959*, a book of prose and poetry. In the book, Wieners, who is described as both gay and bisexual, referred to many drugs and their effects, including "Benzedrine flushes" and later contemplates that he might "regain the right of my mind which Benzedrine may have destroyed. Lost."

Other poets of that time also referred to uppers. In his 1968 work, *Taylor Mead on Amphetamine and in Europe*, Mead describes himself as "a rather famous (or infamous) 'beat generation' poet," a "simple infamous faggot," and a "sissy narcotics addict." Mead, who was the subject of the 1964 Andy Warhol film *Taylor Mead's Ass*, opened the three-hundred-page poem, subtitled *Excerpts from the Anonymous Diary of a New York Youth*, with a preface that read, "This big husky blond young man said 'drink' and I drank this amphetamine in a little teeny glass of water—that was all you Narcos— couldn't be helped—turned me on 48 hours (somewhere in book here is writings)."

This impressive use of speed by Americans from all walks of life is all the more remarkable when one considers that the negative effects of the drugs were noted almost as soon as they entered the marketplace in the 1930s. While studies in 1936 and 1937 noted some unpleasant side effects of Benzedrine use, in 1938 Dr. Benjamin Apfelberg published details of what may be the first reported case of "Benzedrine Sulfate Poisoning," as he termed it, in an article in the *Journal of the American Medical Association.*

The prior year, a twenty-nine-year-old elevator operator was brought to a local New York City hospital unconscious. The man had obtained a prescription for twenty-five ten-milligram Benzedrine sulfate pills after complaining of "depression, exhaustion, and frequent belching." He, apparently, had consumed fourteen of those pills over the course of just a few hours. Apfelberg thought it may have been a suicide attempt. "For the past two years he relates that he had been depressed because of anxiety over his practice of masturbation, which he believed was drying up his brain and skin," Apfelberg wrote. "At first he admitted that he took the overdose of Benzedrine sulfate because he wanted to die, but later he changed his story, insisting that he thought the more he took the sooner he would obtain relief from his gastric symptoms."

Apfelberg noted that this case suggested that "Benzedrine sulfate may become lethal, at least in certain individuals, in far smaller doses than those computed by experimental ratios deducted by its effects on animals."

Also in 1938, Dr. Sidney P. Waud reported in the medical association's journal that he had given "toxic doses" of Benzedrine to a twenty-seven-year-old man on eight separate occasions, eight to ten days apart, to measure the drug's effect on the body. Waud noted a range of symptoms, among them "marked mental depression and general fatigue" that was "constantly present for from three to four days," following the

Benzedrine use. "A definite tolerance of the body for Benzedrine is slowly built up, and increasing doses are necessary to produce the original effects," Waud wrote. "The question of addiction to Benzedrine is not settled, but I believe the possibility is not to be treated lightly for most drugs that produce a pleasant effect on the body (either stimulating or quieting in nature) have their addicts."

Waud described Benzedrine as a drug that was "in common use today and frequently is taken without medical supervision. The Benzedrine Inhaler has been used extensively in infections of the upper respiratory tract." Waud warned that "the indiscriminate use of Benzedrine is very unwise." Other studies, some from as early as 1937, showed that Benzedrine could cause cardiac problems.

While the AMA endorsed Benzedrine in the treatment of narcolepsy and "postencephalitic parkinsonism" in 1937, its Council on Pharmacy and Chemistry noted that the drug "was not recommended for developing a sense of increased energy or capacity." The statement came after students at the University of Minnesota used speed as a study aid. The drug was being used in a study there on the psychological effects of amphetamine.

Smith, in his 1969 study, cited "Pep Teasers," a 1940 article published in *Hygeia*, a health magazine for lay people published by the AMA. The author, Iago Galdston, wrote that "a number of Benzedrine addicts, students, truck drivers, executives, doctors, nurses, and others on prolonged stretches of duty were taking 'pep sniffs.' The results of over addiction are headaches, dizziness, 'jitters,' sleeplessness, and a long train of symptoms frequently ending in grave nervous disorders."

During the 1930s, 1940s, and 1950s, psychosis caused by amphetamine use was repeatedly reported in the scientific literature with the very first such study coming in 1938. It documented three North American cases of psychosis associated with Benzedrine use in men, ages twenty-four, twenty-five, and thirty-eight, and noted another three in other research. The authors reported that the men had experienced paranoia, delusions, and auditory hallucinations.

In 1958, Phillip H. Connell, a researcher in England published *Amphetamine Psychosis*, a monograph that described forty-two cases. By 1968, Connell had documented 201 cases of amphetamine psychosis in the scientific literature.

Reports of amphetamine induced psychosis continued into the 1970s. While many researchers thought the disorder appeared in users who were predisposed toward psychosis, a 1969 study and two 1970 studies showed that the symptoms could occur in people who were not psychotic, but used meth.

Beginning in the mid-1960s, the possibility that chronic amphetamine use may cause brain damage emerged and, over time, a "growing body of evidence is accruing which suggests that intravenous use of amphetamines may cause permanent or long-term brain damage," Spotts and Spotts wrote in *Use and Abuse of Amphetamine and Its Substitutes*.

The cycle of depression leading to more crystal use, which, in turn, causes depression was noted by 1968. "The withdrawal period is characteristically a time of depression, both psychic and physical, and this depression probably reinforces the drive to continue the drug," Seevers wrote in *Amphetamine Abuse*.

The 1960s also saw the emergence of the view that methamphetamine, crime, and violence were linked. Just as there is no evidence today, other than anecdotes, that proves this association, there was no data to support that assertion in the 1960s.

In 1980, Spotts and Spotts wrote, "Reports of incidents of violence and aggression by amphetamine abusers permeate the research literature" and added, "Despite the frequent references to violence and aggression in the amphetamine research literature, there is a paucity of hard or factual information in this area."

Speed was also associated with cheating in sports though that seemed to have little impact on the drug's popularity. Beginning in the 1940s, there were repeated doping scandals in horse racing and professional sports as athletes and trainers took ephedrine or amphetamine, thinking it would give them a competitive edge. "The use of amphetamines in athletics is more widespread than is generally admitted," Seevers wrote. "In the past they have been used extensively for 'doping' race horses, but there is no substantial proof of efficacy in this 'doped' situation." Such doping scandals have continued to today with some professional baseball players being accused of using not just steroids to improve their performance, but also amphetamine.

While the 1960s marked the height of speed use by Americans, that decade also saw a dramatic shift in government's response to speed as well as the medical and popular perception of the drug. Where speed had been celebrated, it was now seen as destructive. Uppers joined such drugs as marijuana, heroin, and opium—three drugs that had long been attacked in the United States that were the subject of a crackdown by state and local governments.

The first federal efforts at controlling illegal drug use date to 1914 when the Harrison Act, which regulated opium, cocaine, and similar products, was passed. At the time, Congress believed that it lacked the legal authority to outlaw the possession of drugs so the act required that anyone who imported, produced, or dealt in these drugs to register with the federal government and pay a tax on any sales. Enforcement of the Harrison Act was given to the Internal Revenue Service. The Harrison Act, however, limited government oversight to only those substances listed in the law. Speed was not listed in the act. While cocaine, the opiates, and later, marijuana, would continue to be subject to state and federal government regulation and criminal laws, uppers were largely exempt for decades.

In 1954, Congress amended the federal Food, Drug, and Cosmetics Act by requiring a prescription for barbiturates and amphetamines. It also gave the U.S. Department of Health, Education, and Welfare the authority to designate drugs as habit forming and requiring a prescription. A violation was a misdemeanor punishable by one year in jail, a $1,000 fine, or both.

The earliest significant federal efforts at attacking speed came in 1955, when Boggs, the congressman from Louisiana, held hearings titled, "Traffic In, and Control of, Narcotics, Barbiturates, and Amphetamines." Four years earlier, Congress had passed the Boggs Act, which set mandatory minimum sentences of two-, five-, and ten-year sentences for first-, second-, and third-time violators of the Harrison Act. It also barred suspended sentences or probation for second- and third-time offenders. At his 1955 hearings, Boggs wanted to determine "the effect which . . . the so-called Boggs law, has had on narcotics traffic."

Boggs was pleased to learn from Harry J. Anslinger, commissioner of narcotics at the Bureau of Narcotics of the U.S. Department of the Treasury that before the Boggs Act passed the average sentence was eighteen months, meaning an offender would serve roughly one third of his sentence. After the Boggs Act, the average sentence was forty-three months.

However, if Boggs thought he was going to draw barbiturates and amphetamines into a similar legal scheme, he must have been disappointed. He held hearings across the country, but his witnesses rarely identified speed as a problem.

The federal government had been operating two drug treatment hospitals for years. One, in Kentucky, had opened in 1935 and the second, in Texas, opened in 1938. Dr. G. Halsey Hunt, assistant surgeon general and associate chief of the Bureau of Medical Services of the U.S. Public Health Service, which operated the hospitals, presented data that showed that no amphetamine users had been treated at the two facilities in 1953 through 1955. Hunt demurred when asked if federal law should be changed to allow speed users to be treated at the two hospitals.

"I think we would have a very serious question about including amphetamine, because it is our present belief, on the basis of what information we have, that the use of amphetamine is one that must be controlled locally," Hunt said. "There is no addiction to amphetamine in the sense of physical dependence, and we do not think that hospitalization for the treatment of amphetamine users would be very effective."

Similarly, a colleague, Congressman J. Arthur Younger of California, had offered a bill that would impose the death penalty on those who sold narcotics, including marijuana, to minors. Would he include barbiturates and amphetamines? "I would not want to do that because, so far as I know, that is not the road which the youngsters take in becoming drug addicts," Younger said. "From my information, practically all of our cases here start with marijuana."

There was only some law enforcement activity related to uppers in 1955. Following a yearlong undercover operation, the FDA and the U.S. Department of Justice announced a joint effort "to stamp out the illegal sale of stimulant drugs to truck drivers by cafes, service stations, truck stops, and drugstores."

U.S. attorneys in ten federal districts and six states simultaneously filed "twenty-two criminal actions and requested bench warrants for the arrest of forty-three individual defendants." The cases alleged violations of the federal Food, Drug, and Cosmetics Act in Virginia, North and South Carolina, Georgia, Illinois, and Indiana.

Altogether, in the 1955 federal fiscal year, 300 criminal cases related to speed, involving over 700 violations, were referred to the justice department by the FDA. Sentences in those cases ranged from three to ten months with an average fine of $500.

The press was beginning to take notice of speed. The Boggs committee staff placed a four-part series by the *St. Louis Globe-Democrat* on "thrill pills" into the hearing record. Part one was titled "Goof Ball Habit Has Become Menace Among Teenagers Here."

In his hearings, Daniel, the senator from Texas, had better luck unearthing anti-speed views during his 1955 hearings, titled "Illicit Narcotics Traffic." A few witnesses reported that speed was a problem though a minor one. The testimony by Dr. John Schultz, chief psychiatrist at the District of Columbia General Hospital, was typical. "Then there is a third group, where it is mostly a matter of abuse, and here we have juveniles, particularly," he said. "They use it for thrills. They combine it very often with Benzedrine, of course, to keep them awake and the barbiturates to give them a feeling of stimulation and benefits they are seeking. Very often it is connected with accidents and sex instances and many other difficulties they get into."

George P. Larrick, the FDA commissioner, presented data on series of cases against pharmacists for the illegal sale of amphetamines. "I want you to go into a little more detail on the amphetamines because this is the first evidence we have had from an official on the subject," Daniel said. The two then held a long discussion on amphetamine use among truck drivers and young people.

"I should say that the amphetamine problem as it relates particularly to kid parties is a sporadic sort of thing," Larrick said. "For a while we had a real trouble spot in New Orleans. At the moment I think that is sort of easing up. We had a lot of trouble in Waco, Houston, San Antonio, your Mexican population also gave us a lot of trouble. We worked closely with the police and the state people and I would not say we cured it any place, but it is somewhat under control."

The real drama came when the two moved on to the case of Carl Austin Hall. In September 1953, Hall and Bonnie Emily Heady had kidnapped and killed six-year-old Bobby Greenlease. They had sought $600,000 in ransom for Greenlease from his father who was a wealthy car dealer. The couple was caught, tried. and executed by December of that year. In his cell on death row, Hall signed a statement that he had been under the influence of Benzedrine during the crime. Larrick put that statement in the hearing record. "We have in our records a signed statement by the murderer that he took amphetamines to gather the courage to commit the murder and to kidnap the child, first, and later to commit the murder," he said.

Not every witness was impressed by the Hall statement. When the subcommittee held hearings in Texas, Owen W. Kilday, the Bexar County sheriff, was asked about amphetamine use in San Antonio. Kilday noted that some jailed inmates had obtained Benzedrine from a doctor's bag that was mistakenly left within their reach. "They didn't go to sleep, raised sand all night," Kilday said. "I think that is getting widespread. I don't think there is too much harm in those drugs."

C. Aubrey Gasque, the subcommittee counsel, was shocked and responded, "Well, the committee has received some evidence that it can be quite harmful." Kilday grew more adamant. "No drug is extremely harmful unless it is a derivative of opium," he said. "That is the threat to the American youth."

Gasque then used the ultimate weapon, the killing of a six-year-old by an amphetamine-fueled murderer. "In Washington, the subcommittee received a statement signed by Bobby Greenlease's murderer to the effect that he was on amphetamines when he killed Bobby Greenlease," he said. Kilday was unmoved. "You come back to the same thing," he said. "He was a criminal who didn't have the nerve to do it. He took that to get the nerve. That drug didn't cause him to do it."

Their hearings were a bust as far as barbiturates and amphetamines were concerned, but Boggs told the *New York Times* in 1955 that while those drugs were "every bit as serious if not more serious" as narcotics there was insufficient information about their use and so legislation could not be drafted to regulate them.

The FDA moved forward in 1959 with a ban on inhalers, but it proved ineffective. The Benzedrine Inhaler had been pulled off the market by Smith, Kline & French Laboratories in 1949, but other products, such as the Dristan and Wyamine inhalers, quickly replaced it. That happened again in 1959 because that ban applied only to inhalers that contained amphetamine so companies continued to produce inhalers with other types of speed such as methamphetamine. One Midwestern company responded by producing and selling an inhaler, named Valo, that contained 150 milligrams of meth. Valo became a very popular product among meth injectors. The FDA restricted their sales to by prescription only in 1965.

Any efforts to demonize speed were dealt a mild blow in 1959 when the AMA released the results of a two-year study that found that speed improved the performance of athletes. Doctors from the Harvard University Medical School and Springfield College in Massachusetts had studied fifty-seven swimmers, runners, or "weight throwers," who given either uppers or a placebo. The athletes who took "large doses of amphetamines" several hours before competing "resulted in a definite performance improvement," the *New York Times* reported. The study results were published in the association's journal, which also condemned the use of speed by athletes.

The year before, Leake published *The Amphetamines: Their Actions and Uses*, a book that can only be described as a spirited defense of speed. "Gradually, as experience with the amphetamines has ripened, they have become firmly established as versatile and helpful remedies, given to millions of people, and under such conditions as to offer remarkably low potential for causing harm or unwanted effects," he wrote. The drug was "subject to distortion by ignorance of their demonstrable actions and successful uses, and by unwise expression of opinion for the sake of publicity, or resulting from prejudice or political expediency." Then Leake warned that "legislation that would interfere with the proper use in medicine of drugs as valuable as the amphetamines would be detrimental to both physicians and to the public."

Efforts by politicians and government agencies to regulate speed and to stigmatize to it were failing. But 1960 saw the first in a series of episodes of amphetamine use that were perceived as epidemics similar to what Japan had witnessed following World War II. Studies on these outbreaks made it clear that the language used to describe speed and the perception of the drug had shifted dramatically since Americans used 50 million Benzedrine Inhalers in 1935 or Mrs. Murphy got a lift from her spiked Ovaltine. What had been pleasurable was now associated with crime or an undesirable counterculture.

In San Francisco, in 1959, only a "few hundred ampules of Methedrine were distributed," Rawlin wrote in *Amphetamine Abuse*. In 1960, that number rose to 280,000, then 580,000 in 1961, and 550,000 between January 1, 1962, and July 17 of that year. In 1963, Burroughs Wellcome stopped the distribution of Methedrine in California pharmacies at the request of that state's Board of Pharmacy and attorney general. Other pharmaceutical companies that made injectable amphetamine products did the same.

Spotts and Spotts described two "mini-amphetamine epidemics," one in St. Louis, Missouri in the early 1960s, which was "apparently caused by a heroin shortage," and the second in Washington, D.C., in 1972 and was also caused by a heroin shortage.

Publishing in *Amphetamine Abuse*, Dr. John D. Griffith, a professor in the psychiatry department at Vanderbilt University's School of Medicine, reported on amphetamine abuse in Oklahoma City in 1966. He noted that one of the local graduate students hired to work on the study turned out to be a user. "This was first suspected when, after being asked to comment on a minor research project, he turned out a 453-page book which was largely unintelligible," Griffith wrote.

The big outbreak came in Haight-Ashbury in 1968. In 1967, during the Summer of Love in San Francisco, the popular drug had been LSD, according to one study in *Use and Abuse of*

Amphetamine and Its Substitutes, but by early 1968 amphetamine was the dominant drug there and the users were predominantly white and young as well as mixed male and female.

Meth was so bad that the hippies, the symbol of the 1960s
counterculture, had rejected it, according to Ellinwood.
"Even the hippies have noted the dangerous aspects of
amphetamine abuse in their slogan 'Speed Kills,'" he wrote.

In a further indication of how far speed had come since
Harry the Hipster had sung about it, Smith titled his 1969
study of meth use in Haight-Ashbury, "The Marketplace of
Speed: Compulsive Methamphetamine Abuse and Violence"
and a second rendition of the same data published in Spotts
and Spotts's "Compulsive Methamphetamine Abuse and
Criminality in the Haight-Ashbury District."

Medical terms were now being applied regularly to speed
use. It was an epidemic or an outbreak though how these epidemics differed from the explosive growth in amphetamine
use in other parts of American society was never explained by
these authors.

The pharmaceutical industry and doctors would soon be
accused of being one more criminal element in the speed culture. That began in 1962, when the FDA, under Larrick,
released its study, estimating that 4.5 billion ten-milligram
amphetamine doses were produced annually in America and
half of them were diverted to illegal uses.

The FDA offered no supporting evidence for its assertion
concerning the diversion of billions of pills, but politicians
and public figures would continue to cite that statistic for the
next decade even after the federal Bureau of Narcotics and
Dangerous Drugs produced its own study in 1967 that estimated that just 16 percent of all legally produced amphetamines and barbiturates were "unaccounted for."

In 1962, President John F. Kennedy supported stronger controls on these drugs. "Society's gains will be illusory if we reduce the incidence of one kind of drug dependency, only to have new kinds of drugs substituted," he said. "The use of these drugs is increasing problems of abnormal and social behavior, highway accidents, juvenile delinquency, and broken homes."

Kennedy established his Advisory Commission on Narcotic and Drug Abuse in 1963, which recommended stricter controls on prescription drugs.

Congress once again entered the fight in 1964 when the Senate Subcommittee on Health of the Committee on Labor and Public Welfare held hearings on the "Control of Psychotoxic Drugs." Larrick was a featured witness.

While barbiturates and amphetamines had "a wide range of usefulness," these drugs were "subject to widespread abuses" and "their non-medical use has contributed to the rising toll of deaths on our highways, juvenile delinquency, and promiscuity, and violent and bizarre crimes," he said. "An otherwise law abiding citizen may go berserk under the influence of psycho-toxic drugs and become a menace to himself and society; he may participate in mass violence while abusing the drugs; and, it is not uncommon for hoodlums who are planning a robbery or other criminal acts to take amphetamines to bolster their courage."

Earlier laws passed by Congress were "no longer adequate to prevent widespread illegal sale of the drugs" and Larrick called for "adequate control over drugs which cannot be proved to have passed in interstate commerce, adequate provisions to restrict these drugs to the legitimate channels of prescription drugs, adequate recordkeeping and inventory controls, and prohibitions against possession by persons for non-medical use and distribution."

Faced with new recordkeeping requirements and clearly resenting any implication that they were complicit in the illegal distribution of these drugs, industry groups, to varying degrees, resisted any new legislation. Ralph R. Rooke, chairman of the Committee on Legislation of the National Association of Retail Druggists, told the subcommittee that his organization opposed the bill because it gave FDA authority to inspect prescription files of pharmacies without a warrant and if that provision were eliminated his group would back the bill. The FDA was "intent on grabbing new and broader authority," Rooke said.

W. Roy Smith, chairman of the Committee on Legislation of the American Pharmaceutical Association, agreed with Rooke and added that his organization was concerned about the costs of the recordkeeping requirements. When Smith noted that the majority of pharmacists were law abiding, Senator Ralph W. Yarborough of Texas pointed out that during the ten-year period ending December 31, 1962, 1,658 firms or individuals were convicted of the illegal sale of barbiturates and amphetamines and "78 percent were retail drug firms, pharmacists, or their employees." The most vehement opposition came from the AMA, which wrote in a July 31, 1964, letter to the subcommittee that "the proposed bill is restrictive to the degree that it would inhibit and interfere with the legitimate manufacture, distribution and use of these drugs."

The opposition lost. In 1965, the Drug Abuse Control Amendments were enacted. They required more recordkeeping by manufacturers, wholesalers, doctors, pharmacists, and retail outlets and made possession of certain drugs, including amphetamines, by anyone other than the ultimate user with a prescription illegal. The amendments exempted over–the-counter products and certain other drugs deemed non–habit forming. The law was amended in 1968 to add criminal penalties for the illegal possession and sale of the covered drugs. At least twenty-eight states enacted laws similar to the Drug Abuse Control Amendments in 1965 and 1966, Daniel W. Byles, the corporate counsel at Merck and Company, wrote in *Amphetamine Abuse*.

The pharmaceutical industry was stung not so much by the loss, but by the rhetorical salvos that were being directed at it from Capitol Hill. In *Amphetamine Abuse*, Margarita C. Russell, a senior literature scientist at Smith, Kline & French Laboratories, defended the industry. "Today, the public probably has more confidence in its physicians and the drugs that they use than ever before," Russell wrote. "Undeserved criticism of the medical and allied professions coupled with sensational reports of the horrors of drugs, however, can completely destroy this confidence. Reputable manufacturers should not be accused of the misguided and illegal transactions of fly-by-night companies operating under the umbrella of the industry or those who run strictly illegal operations."

Congress was not finished with the industry. By 1971, a House report characterized the 1965 amendments as a "failure" and one of the primary reasons for that was the pharmaceutical manufacturers.

The report was generated from testimony taken during a series of 1969 hearings held around the nation by the House Select Committee on Crime. The committee chair, Congressman Claude Pepper of Florida, led an assault on the industry. The committee had subpoenaed sales records from a number of amphetamine manufacturers. The theory was that the manufacturers were selling large quantities of amphetamines and barbiturates to wholesalers in the Southwest who were, in turn, selling them to companies in Mexico. In some cases, the manufacturers sold directly to Mexican companies. The drugs were then smuggled back into the United States. and sold illegally. The committee called the heads of those companies in to testify.

Coe from Burroughs Wellcome was accompanied by William F. Dowling, the company's general counsel, and Kathryn V. Crean, an assistant counsel. "Are you aware that some of your products have been seized at the Mexican border?" Richard W. Kurrus, chief counsel for the committee, asked Coe.

"I was not aware of that until today," Coe responded. Kurrus then asked Coe to read seizure data into the record.

"'1968. Burroughs Wellcome product, Methedrine, units seized, twelve hundred,'" Coe said. "I do not know if that is tablets or injection or bottles or what. I have never seen these figures before, sir."

Moments later, Kurrus pressed Coe on the seizure data. "Let me ask you this," he said. "Is it fair to say that a significant percentage of your products get into the illegal market, not, certainly, through your fault, but, unfortunately, that this does occur?"

Coe responded, "I would not say, in my opinion, that a significant part do. As far as I am aware, I think there are some, yes."

Donald K. Fletcher, manager of distribution at Smith, Kline & French Laboratories was joined by Clifford C. Davis, the company's legislative counsel. They received harsher treatment than Coe as Pepper came close to accusing the company of knowingly participating in smuggling. "Now, do you think there is any good reason why your sales to Mexico have increased, more than doubled, since 1960?" Pepper asked. "Could the inference be properly drawn that the southwestern part of the United States is a conduit of these dangerous drug that have to be sold under licenses into Mexico which, given the considerable increase in the volume of these drugs to Mexico, is perhaps becoming a source of supply in the black market to places in the United States?"

Fletcher responded, "Mr. Chairman, I would like to say that I have already recognized the fact that we know that small quantities of our products are available in pharmacies in Mexico. We do not believe and no one has ever shown me any indication that these products are available from our customers, the wholesalers."

Irving C. Udell, president of Bates Laboratories, and Richard C. Calkins, Udell's counsel, was humiliated.

Kurrus read a series of Bates's invoices that were sent to an address in Mexico. The company had shipped 15 million pills to that address "during the last few years." The committee staff had visited that address and, as Udell sat at the witness table, Kurrus disclosed that if it were an actual address, it would be the fourteenth hole of a golf course in Tijuana. The committee staff had also tipped the Bureau of Narcotics and Dangerous Drugs, which promptly seized 1.2 million uppers shipped by Bates that were on their way to that location.

For Pepper, the stakes were very high.

"The destruction of our youth, through dangerous drug abuse, does not involve merely the destruction of an isolated thrill seeker or a disillusioned person who has succumbed to the use of such drugs, such destruction vitally affects the victim's family, his friends, the community, and the nation," he said. "In many ways, our society has unleashed a Frankenstein-type monster over which we seemingly have no control."

The response was tougher laws.

"Our laws have not been adequate to deal with this fantastic problem, nor have they kept pace with it," Pepper said. "[T]here are no meaningful or adequate controls on the exportation of these dangerous drugs . . . [T]here is no adequate control, federal or state control, over the purchase of the immediate precursors or chemical ingredients needed to manufacture these dangerous drugs, particularly LSD and methamphetamines."

That tougher law was the Comprehensive Drug Abuse Prevention and Control Act of 1970. It required manufacturers, distributors, and dispensers of these drugs to register with the justice department and placed even more stringent record-keeping and reporting requirements on the drugs.

It allowed drugs to be moved quickly from a loosely controlled status, Schedule V, to the controls that grew increasingly stringent under Schedules IV through I. Schedule I drugs, such as LSD or heroin, have no medical use and a high potential for abuse. In 1971, amphetamines were made Schedule II drugs.

In addition to placing even greater controls on speed, the government would now set annual production quotas on uppers that correspond with medical needs. One 1973 study put the 1972 legal production of amphetamine base at twenty thousand pounds, which was roughly equivalent to 20 percent of the production in 1971. The law also regulated the precursor chemicals used to make amphetamines and barbiturates.

The federal government had won the speed war. It also created an entirely new problem that Larrick had effectively predicted in 1955 when testifying before the Daniel subcommittee. "Have you had any bootleg production of amphetamines and barbiturates?" Daniel asked the FDA commissioner. "I am not aware of such production," Larrick said. "We are aware of smuggling from Mexico. We have an occasional problem of smuggling from abroad. Today the pressures against illegal sales have probably not been great enough in this country to drive the thing underground as it will be underground more and more as we bring the pressures on the problem."

It did not take long for that "underground" to arrive. In his 1969 study, Smith wrote that the first known meth labs started up in the San Francisco area in the early 1960s. They appeared after police and state regulatory agencies cracked down on the meth use there. "[S]peed labs began to operate as early as 1962, and by 1963 several labs were in operation in the San Francisco Bay Area," Smith wrote. "Because of the shortage of speed in other cities on the West Coast, the manufacture and distribution of speed became an extremely profitable enterprise."

Drug labs quickly spread across the country and, in 1967, the New York City newspapers reported that agents from the federal Bureau of Drug Abuse Control had raided one lab just two blocks from City Hall in downtown Manhattan. Agents seized a pound and a half of meth.

The next year, *Look* magazine ran a long story, titled "The Cruel Chemical World of Speed," that told readers that "federal agents have busted labs from Chicago to Santa Cruz, Calif., and grabbed fifty pounds on Long Island."

A 1981 U.S. General Accounting Office report that weighed the effectiveness of the DEA's anti-drug efforts noted that despite the "impressive increase in the number of clandestine laboratory seizures—234 in 1980 compared to 33 in 1975—clandestine laboratories continue to flourish." In each of those six years, the majority of those labs were producing amphetamine or methamphetamine with 147 out of 237 making speed in 1979 and 146 out of 234 manufacturing uppers in 1980.

A 1988 GAO report found that from 1981 to 1986, the number of meth lab seizures went from 89 to 412 and amphetamine lab seizures went from 14 to 63. Similarly, meth-related emergency room visits and deaths rose from 1983 to 1986 while such visits and deaths for other "dangerous drugs" fell in that period.

In 1988, 1993, and 1996, the federal government responded by increasing the regulation of the precursor chemicals used to manufacture crystal as well as the over-the-counter drugs that contain ephedrine and pseudoephedrine. While the federal government claimed that these efforts had some initial success, the recent growth in small toxic labs suggests that the manufacturers have managed to stay ahead of the DEA.

The more serious change came in the late 1980s and early 1990s when Mexican crime organizations moved into the meth business. "A second development reported by law enforcement agencies has been the apprehension of illegal aliens hired by organized groups of criminals to produce methamphetamine and initiate distribution," wrote Miller and Dr. Bruce Heischober, an assistant professor of adolescent and emergency medicine at Loma Linda University Medical Center School of Medicine, in a 1991 monograph published by the National Institute on Drug Abuse.

Throughout the 1990s and into the twenty-first century, the DEA would continue to note that the U.S. meth business was now dominated by these crime groups. These organizations had several advantages over the small labs. They could relocate their manufacturing on the Mexican side of the border where they are beyond the reach of U.S. laws and subject to enforcement that was less than rigorous. They had preexisting distribution networks that moved cocaine and other drugs and they produced a better product.

Some gay and bisexual men were their customers.

In their monograph, Miller and Heischober wrote that, in San Francisco and the four surrounding counties, amphetamine use was cited in just 4 percent of the drug-treatment admissions from 1986 through the first half of 1990, but gay men were most of the users. "Gays (homosexual men) in their twenties and thirties accounted for a predominate number of methamphetamine abusers in this area," the authors wrote.

In Los Angeles, Miller and Heischober noted that meth use was low except in that city's gay enclave. "[I]n the West Hollywood area there is a much higher prevalence of methamphetamine abuse," they wrote. "This is also an area with a predominantly gay population. In conversations with physicians and substance abuse counselors in this area and in the Bay area of San Francisco, Heischober learned that methamphetamine is preferred by gays because it allegedly has the ability to enhance and prolong sexual performance."

Several studies published in the mid- to late 1990s documented speed use, including injection use, among gay men in Seattle and elsewhere in the West. "Because of the commonly reported aphrodisiacal effects of methamphetamines, study of users' sexual behaviors may be particularly relevant," wrote E. Michael Gorman, a professor at the University of Washington, in a 1997 study published in the *Medical Anthropology Quarterly*. "At least in part because of such properties, the drug (known commonly as 'speed,' 'crystal,' or 'crank') has gained considerable popularity among gay and bisexual men."

As the 1999 NYU center study shows, meth soon made its across the country. "This project came out of my concern over the last several years about the growing number of incidents of crystal use that I was seeing," Halkitis said in 2000 when the study, dubbed Project Tina, was released. The rapid recruitment for Project Tina was significant. "It tells me that it is popular," Halkitis said. "It's a growing problem. The fact that we recruited fifty guys in forty-eight days says that."

In New York City, in 2000, there was an awareness on the street that crystal had arrived. In an interview outside the Big Cup with *Lesbian and Gay New York* about why some gay men had not gone to the Millennium March on Washington, a political event produced by the Human Rights Campaign, the nation's largest gay lobbying group, Doug, a thirty-seven-year-old, gay man, said bitterly, "There's just no interest in it. There's no crystal meth involved." Crystal had arrived.

Methamphetamine had gone from being a near wonder drug to some physicians, Mrs. Murphy's pick-me-up, and a tool for soldiers and pilots to a drug that created addicts and was associated with violence and crime. The language used to talk about speed had shifted as well. Where its widespread use was detected, this was no longer "having fun and going on forever," but an "epidemic" or an "outbreak." Speed had been pulled out of the popular culture and placed under the control of medicine and the law.

As this shift took place, gay men, like millions of Americans, were using many forms of speed, including meth and those gay men were drawn into that new understanding of the drug. Their speed use was now a medical problem and, to an extent, a legal problem that had to be addressed by law enforcement.

This shift did not necessarily have to occur among in the gay community, but one thing made it more likely that it would. Those community groups that had traditionally served the gay men with HIV prevention and health services had been struggling for years to assist their clients. That core group of gay men who used drugs, including crystal, and had unsafe sex had gone largely unaddressed.

Instead, the community had been distracted by a series of often bitter debates over the regulation of bathhouses and sex clubs, the role that oral sex might play in the spread of HIV, and even whether or not the AIDS epidemic among gay men had ended.

As more gay men began to use meth, researchers and a just few AIDS groups took note. Crystal use spread largely unchecked and unnoticed in the gay male community.

3

ENDLESS TALKING ABOUT ENDLESS FUCKING

Some 300 people had pressed into the main hall of New York City's Lesbian and Gay Community Services Center on a cold November evening in 1994.

This was years before the center was remodeled and took on a new, more inclusive name, but that room, with its low ceiling and poor lighting, was home to the gay community. It had hosted the Monday night meetings of ACT UP and countless town hall events where issues of concern to the gay and lesbian community were debated and discussed.

On this evening, the crowd was driven by the view that there was a resurgence of unsafe sex among gay men and they had come to hear a panel discussion with the chilling title "Are We Surviving: The State of HIV Prevention in the Gay and Lesbian Communities." The answer from the panelists was "no."

San Francisco psychologist Walt Odets described the bleak state of the HIV prevention efforts at that time. "There's no question that prevention has failed," Odets said.

His book *In the Shadow of the Epidemic: Being HIV-Negative in the Age of AIDS* was published in 1995 and, in his book, Odets argued that HIV prevention had failed to distinguish between gay and bisexual men who were HIV-negative and those who were HIV-positive. The needs of those two populations were very different.

While Odets was criticized for basing his work on the small number of men he counseled in his therapy practice and for an excessive emphasis on the role that survivor guilt might be playing in leading men to have unsafe sex, his message was seen as important. It was a point he made on that November evening.

"Primary prevention has to name the population it wants to keep uninfected," he said, suggesting a radical, and controversial, departure from past prevention practices.

AIDS prevention messages had not weighed the needs and experience of HIV-negative men specifically, choosing instead to broadcast a generic "play safe" theme tailored to avoid offending men who were HIV-positive. Other language in the AIDS liturgy seemed to dangerously minimize the impact of HIV and failed to state plainly that being HIV-negative is better than being HIV-positive.

"If men are 'thriving,' 'living with AIDS,' or 'long-term survivors' then what was so wrong with being HIV-positive?" Odets said.

Speaking of a community that was well into its thirteenth year of the AIDS epidemic, Robin Miller, GMHC's director of evaluation research and another panelist, said, "There is little agreement about criteria for successful prevention" and added later, "We must decide what we mean by prevention."

These were remarkable statements given that many in the lesbian and gay community routinely credited safe sex with having dramatically reduced HIV prevalence, or the percentage who are infected, and HIV incidence, or the percentage who are newly infected in a year, among gay men. HIV prevalence and incidence among those men had reached horrifying heights in the 1980s. Those numbers were made possible by the sprawling sexual landscape that gay men created in the late 1970s and early 1980s.

In the decades prior to the arrival of HIV, gay men sought out one another for sex and intimacy in a variety of public venues. They risked assault, arrest, prosecution, prison, the loss of a job, and many other ills for a moment of pleasure, and sometimes more than that, with another man or men. Such was the strength of their desire. With the rise of the gay movement in the late 1950s culminating in the 1969 riots at the Stonewall Inn in New York City, the community saw growth in businesses that sought to satisfy that desire.

In his 1987 book, *And the Band Played On*, the late Randy Shilts, a San Francisco journalist, estimated that the North American industry serving gay men with "hundreds" of bathhouses, sex clubs, and bars with backrooms was grossing $100 million a year. Major American cities offered gay and bisexual men multiple businesses to choose from with some appealing to particular sexual tastes.

These were not mere sex businesses. Gay men who lived during that time speak of them as places where they had fabulous sex, but also met new friends or lovers, or escaped from a world that was openly hostile toward them.

In his 2003 book, *Stayin' Alive: The Invention of Safe Sex*, Richard Berkowitz described his life as a gay man and a hustler working in New York City in the late 1970s and early 1980s.

"I was making mistakes along the way, but I felt that sex was the way gay men felt more fully alive in a world where so many wanted us eradicated," he wrote.

Berkowitz, along with Dr. Joseph Sonnabend and the late Michael Callen, is credited with the creation and distribution of a 1983 pamphlet, the first of its kind, that discussed the suspected causes of AIDS and taught gay men how to avoid becoming infected by using condoms or engaging in other behaviors that could reduce their risk of infection. For Berkowitz, New York City before AIDS was heaven.

"For me, gay life in New York City before the dawn of AIDS was like living in the Promised Land," Berkowitz wrote. "Whatever fantasy you had, you always knew you could satisfy it any time, night or day, at one of the many sexual playgrounds . . . Although it often seemed like sex was becoming the only glue that held gay men together, sex often led to enduring friendships and even relationships; but it was hard staying focused on one person for long when you were living in a bustling sexual amusement park."

For some, sex between men was part of sexual liberation, a political philosophy that sought to remove the social and legal constraints on sexual expression. In that philosophy, the sex was an act of defiance at a time when there were still sodomy laws on the books that were actively enforced and it was the ultimate statement of "gay is good."

The sex also offered a respite from the battle. The community's political struggle for equality was proceeding, at best, slowly. The bathhouses and sex clubs were places to escape from that fight and the anti-gay bigotry that the community still confronts. Defeats in that struggle were all too common.

Publishing in the *Village Voice* in 1982, the late Arthur Bell wrote, "A common attitude of the gay on the street is 'Fuck them all. I'll live my life without it,'" referring to a New York City law that banned discrimination based on sexual orientation that had been voted down in the City Council for the tenth time in as many years. Bell continued, "The gay-on-the-run has given up on politics, organizations, zaps, and formal gay liberation. Liberation in the 1980s is internal. Check Saturday night at the Saint."

Some gay men were taking full advantage of the sexual landscape that was available to them. Berkowitz quoted Callen speaking to a group of doctors in 1982 saying, "As the National Cancer Institute reported this year, 'The median number of lifetime sexual partners for gay AIDS victims being studied is 1,160.' One thousand, one hundred and sixty! That number indicates a very specific lifestyle."

Callen, who was clearly enjoying discussing his sex life with the doctors, described his own couplings. "I am twenty-seven years old," he said. "I've been having gay sex in the tearooms, bathhouses, bookstores, backrooms, and adult movie theaters since I came out at seventeen. I estimate conservatively that I have had sex with over three thousand different partners."

At that time, Callen believed that AIDS was not caused by a virus, but by the cumulative effect on the immune system of having many sexually transmitted diseases that resulted from having many sexual partners. He cited his experience as evidence to support that theory. Callen was not alone in racking up large numbers of partners.

In his 1997 book, *Sexual Ecology: AIDS and the Destiny of Gay Men*, Gabriel Rotello cited the work of Dr. June Osborn, a researcher at the federal National Institutes of Health, or NIH, who was studying sexually transmitted diseases among gay men and struggling to define multiple sex partners.

"Every time we do an NIH site visit, the definition of 'multiple sex partners' has changed," Rotello quoted Osborn saying in 1980. "First it was twenty partners a year. That was 1975. Then in 1976 it was fifty partners a year. By 1978, we were talking about a hundred sexual partners a year and now we're using the term to describe five hundred partners in a single year."

In an often cited Osborn quote, she said, "I am duly in awe."

Among the consequences of all of this sexual activity were, not surprisingly, many sexually transmitted diseases. Before HIV came on the scene, gay men were contending with syphilis, gonorrhea, herpes, hepatitis A and B, and a host of other infections. When he argued that AIDS was caused by the collapse of the immune system, Callen often listed the many diseases he had experienced.

"From 1973, when I came out to 1975, I only got mononucleosis and nonspecific urethritis, or NSU," Berkowitz quoted Callen saying. "In 1975, I got my first case of gonorrhea. Not bad, I thought. I'd had maybe two hundred different partners and I'd only gotten the clap twice. But then, moving from Boston to New York City, it all began to snowball. First came hepatitis A in 1976 and more gonorrhea and more NSU. In 1977, I was diagnosed with amebiasis, an intestinal parasite, hepatitis B, more gonorrhea, and NSU. In 1978, more amebiasis and my first case of shigella, and of course, more gonorrhea. Then in 1979, hepatitis yet a third time, this time type non-A, non-B, more intestinal parasites, adding giardia this time, and an anal fissure as well as my first case of syphilis. In 1980, the usual gonorrhea, shigella twice, and more amebiasis. By 1981, I got some combination of STDs each and every time I had sex, and I finally contracted herpes."

Callen did not discuss the sexually transmitted diseases he had contended with to condemn gay sex. On the contrary, he was a great defender of that sex even to the point that the 1983 pamphlet he produced with Berkowitz and Sonnabend was titled, "How to Have Sex in an Epidemic:

One Approach," but his experience with these infections was typical of that portion of the gay male community that was highly sexually active.

The data on sexually transmitted diseases from that time often did not distinguish between infections among homosexuals or heterosexuals, who were swapping plenty of these infections, but one type of gonorrhea—rectal gonorrhea in men—is an unambiguous indicator of gay sex.

In 1980, 1,869 cases of male rectal gonorrhea were reported to the New York City health department. That same year, in San Francisco, there were over 5,000 cases of male rectal gonorrhea.

Shilts noted two studies, one from Seattle, Washington and the second from Denver, Colorado, that implicated the sex businesses in the spread of sexually transmitted diseases. The Seattle study found that among gay men who had shigellosis, 69 percent met their sex partners in bathhouses. Similarly, the Denver study concluded that one in eight men who were visiting bathhouses there had asymptomatic syphilis or gonorrhea. With an average 2.7 sex partners per night, a gay man in a Denver bathhouse had a one out of three chance of going home with one or the other infection.

The large number of sexually transmitted diseases among gay men is not merely an indicator of the amount of sex some of these men were having. HIV has evolved to take advantage of such infections by increasing its reproduction when they are present and the virus can use the inflamed tissue or sores caused by some of these diseases to transmit itself between infected and uninfected people. Some studies have estimated that a sexually transmitted disease increases the likelihood of acquiring or transmitting HIV two to five times.

The highly sexually active men became a reservoir where

the virus thrived. HIV prevalence and incidence in that population was very high so any gay man who had sex with one of these men had a good chance of becoming infected even if he tended to have far fewer partners in a year.

With the virus spreading throughout the community of gay men, many of these men were newly infected. One attribute of a new infection is that the person is also highly infectious with a large amount of virus in his blood and semen. As that man has sex with other partners he is much more likely to infect them.

The sheer volume of sex that some gay men were enjoying, the sexually transmitted diseases, and the large amount of HIV that was living in gay male bodies and was available to infect others sent HIV incidence and prevalence among gay men through the roof.

In 2004, Dr. Mary Ann Chiasson, vice president of research and evaluation at the Medical and Health Research Association of New York City, discussed studies that tested stored blood samples to determine the HIV incidence rate among gay and bisexual men in New York City. In 1978, it was 6.6 percent. It increased in later years.

"What they found when they looked at these stored samples was that the annual incidence of sero-conversion was between 5.5 percent and 10.6 percent," Chiasson said. "You can see how the epidemic got started."

Incidence is cumulative so if a population were to sustain an annual incidence rate of 10.6 percent for just three years then 32 percent, or nearly one third of that population, would be infected at the end of that time. HIV incidence rates among some gay men in other American cities were just as high. Given those incidence rates it is easy to see how other studies have estimated that in the late 1970s and 1980s, HIV prevalence among gay men in major American cities ranged from 20 to 50 percent.

These numbers do not begin to describe the horror that the lesbian and gay community lived through during the 1980s. While AIDS was first noted in 1981, the virus was not discovered until 1984. That the cause of the disease was unknown only contributed to the fear that AIDS created in the gay community. Blood tests to detect antibodies to the virus or the virus itself were not widely available for several years. It was often the case that a gay man learned he was infected only when the most severe and life threatening symptoms of the disease appeared.

The first anti-HIV drug, AZT, came on the market in 1987 and there were few drugs available to treat many of the opportunistic infections that are associated with AIDS. It was a common experience to bring a sick friend or lover to the hospital with the understanding that he would die there.

In their 2000 book, *AIDS Doctors: Voices from the Epidemic*, Ronald Bayer and Gerald M. Oppenheimer interviewed roughly eighty doctors who treated people with AIDS in the 1980s and 1990s. Some of those doctors were gay themselves and as frightened as any other gay man.

"We were all going to die," the authors quoted Dr. John Mazzullo saying. "There was no reason why we shouldn't have died."

Mazzullo remained uninfected. A second doctor, Ronald Grossman, described doing an inventory of his body, a common practice among gay men, searching for swollen lymph nodes or other symptoms associated with AIDS.

"I remember the time when I caught myself examining my own lymph nodes with such vigor that I made my own neck sore, and validated that I must have swollen lymph nodes," Grossman said. "I think we were all terrified."

Safe sex provided a tool to combat that terror. In *Stayin'*
Alive, Berkowitz related one of his conversations with Callen
and Sonnabend about the possibility of educating gay men
about condom use or other ways of reducing their risk of
becoming infected.

"I keep running into guys I know on the streets who don't
want to hear a word about AIDS," he said. "They were so terrified, they told me to shut up or they would walk away;
there's no way they would be willing to discuss it before
having sex."

Sonnabend responded, "But that won't last. In the mean-
time one should try to find ways to approach sex safely while
trying to encourage some sort of sexual ethic to promote
responsibility. Different men will require different advice, but
saying that one should stop sex completely suggests that
sexual expression has no value, and that is contradictory to
human nature. Sex is a vital part of being alive."

It was in this conversation that Sonnabend suggested that
promoting condom use could be one way to "interrupt disease
transmission" among gay men. In the midst of this terror, safe
sex was born.

In 1983, Callen and Berkowitz released their pamphlet with
a foreword written by Sonnabend. As the title suggests, the
pamphlet did not attempt to substantially reconfigure the
"bustling sexual amusement park" that Berkowitz had played
in. On the contrary, part of the intent was to preserve that
infrastructure. The authors were explicit in their defense of
gay sex.

"Our challenge is to figure out how we can have gay, life-
affirming sex, satisfy our emotional needs, and stay alive!"
they wrote at the close of their introduction.

The pamphlet, which became the model for later safe sex

campaigns, discussed the relative risks of "disease transmission" through oral and anal sex, made recommendations about when gay men should use condoms, and suggested a range of sexual activities that gay men could engage in that would substantially reduce or eliminate their risk of becoming infected.

Callen and Berkowitz indicted promiscuity and the sex businesses in the spread of diseases. They instructed their readers to limit their partners in these places to one or two and to exercise great caution when they had sex there. That advice bred opposition.

For some in the gay community, the bathhouses and sex clubs were the embodiment of sexual liberation. Promiscuity was the physical expression of a philosophy that rejected all constraints on sexuality. Callen and Berkowitz were attacked by some community leaders and organizations. Berkowitz charged that the American Foundation for AIDS Research, GMHC, and even the CDC were obstructing his efforts.

"[T]hey actively opposed those of us who produced these recommendations with our own resources," he wrote. That would change. It is now commonplace for advocates to point to the reductions in HIV prevalence and incidence as well as risk-taking behaviors among gay and bisexual that were seen in the late 1980s and into the 1990s as evidence of the effectiveness of safe sex campaigns, but the picture is more complex than that assertion suggests.

A major contributor to those reductions was the disease itself. It is a gruesome fact that HIV first made some gay men so sick that they were physically unable to have sex and thereby infect others. Then the disease killed them and ended any possibility that they could transmit the virus to a sex partner.

Some have suggested that fear—the terror that Berkowitz and Grossman referred to—moved gay men to dramatically change their sex practices. Some studies that show changes in behavior among gay men support that view, but one could just as easily look at that data and conclude that those men weighed the information about how HIV is transmitted and made a rational decision to protect themselves not out of fear, but out of self-interest. What is clear is that many gay men changed their behavior. Some of those changes predate the appearance of the first safe sex pamphlet.

A 1987 San Francisco study that followed a group of 125 gay men from 1978 to 1985 reported that the median number of nonsteady partners went from sixteen to one for 90 percent of the men in the group. The median is the number that sits in the middle of a range of numbers so that shift demonstrates a large reduction in the number of partners.

A second San Francisco study, reported in 1985, found that in a group of 454 gay men, the average number of sex partners went from 6.3 to 3.9 between 1982 and 1984 and the men reduced their condomless anal sex by over 50 percent.

A Columbia University study of 746 New York City gay men that was published in 1994 found that the percentage reporting unsafe anal sex, in all age groups, fell dramatically from 1980 through 1991. For the entire group, the average number of unsafe sex contacts went from eleven per year down to one per year.

The Multicenter AIDS Cohort Study, or MACS, which followed nearly 5,000 gay and bisexual men in multiple cities across the country reported that between 1984 and 1986 the number of men who reported being either celibate or in a monogamous relationship went from 14 percent to 39 percent while the number who said they did not have receptive anal sex went from 26 percent to 49 percent during that time.

Some gay men, often with little or no help from government or community groups, were making decisions that were intended to reduce or eliminate their risk of becoming infected with HIV. The adoption of safe-sex practices, however, was incomplete at best and by the early 1990s, AIDS groups and activists, such as Odets, were sounding the alarm.

The Columbia University study concluded that gay men had changed their behavior, but only to the point that they were sitting on the cusp of eventually extinguishing the epidemic or watching it grow. Using a mathematical model, the study estimated that if New York City gay men averaged just one unsafe sex contact per year, as opposed to two or more, the epidemic would end over time though that could take as long as fifty years.

"We found the current sexual behavior of gay men to be right on the epidemic boundary so that HIV potentially could fade out under the right conditions or proliferate if there is even a small increase in unsafe sex," said Laura Dean, one of the study authors, in a 1994 press statement. "The good news is that if safer sex is maintained and infection from other sources like drug injection is prevented, our results indicate that the HIV epidemic could fade out over time."

Other studies showed irregular condom use. A 1994 study in San Francisco reported on the results of a survey of 380 eighteen- to twenty-nine-year-old gay men in that city. Sixty-three percent of those men reported having had one or more partners for receptive anal sex in the prior twelve months and 41 percent of those men did not use condoms consistently. Eighteen percent of the men in sample were already infected. The authors estimated the annual HIV incidence rate in that population at 2.6 percent. While that incidence rate is far lower than those reported in the 1980s, it is high enough to keep the epidemic growing in that population.

This data was being reported out of major cities where community groups had made a concerted effort to disseminate information about safe sex and condom use. In smaller American cities, where gay men had perhaps not benefited from such education programs, the news was also mixed.

In a series of studies published in the late 1980s and early 1990s, Dr. Jeffrey A. Kelly, a professor at the Medical College of Wisconsin and the director of the Center for AIDS Intervention Research, showed that some gay men in smaller cities were having plenty of unsafe sex.

A 1990 study surveyed gay men in "three small southern cities" and found that 24 percent reported having had unprotected anal sex in the prior two months. Among the 24 percent, unprotected anal sex occurred an average of six times during that two-month period. An earlier Kelly study, published in 1988, surveyed gay men in "somewhat larger cities," such as Seattle, Washington and Tampa, Florida, and reported that 37 percent had had unprotected anal sex in the prior six months.

It was the 1992 study by Kelly that shocked the AIDS community. The study surveyed nearly two thousand gay men in "sixteen cities with populations under two hundred thousand in four different regions of the country." Eighty-five percent of the men completed a questionnaire about their sexual practices that was distributed at clubs and bars and nearly one third of those men said that they had had unprotected anal sex an average of eight times in the prior six months.

In one respect, the panelists at that 1994 event were correct. Some gay men were not having safe sex, but the panelists also made a mistake. It was not the case that all gay men had embraced safe sex and were now slipping. A portion of the gay male community had never adopted safe sex. The community only noticed that group in the early 1990s. The news that some gay men were having unsafe sex was only a part of the picture that confronted the audience and panelists during that 1994 event at the gay center.

In June of 1993, data presented at the Ninth International AIDS Conference, held in Berlin, had dispelled any notion that a cure for the disease was even close to being developed. Some in the gay community, perhaps many, had held onto the unrealistic belief that safe sex was a temporary measure that would be used only until HIV could be wiped out.

During the November panel, Richard Elovich, GMHC's director of Substance Use Counseling and Education, said the news out of the Berlin conference was the shattering of "an illusion that we were going to see a cure in our lifetime, that AIDS was going to be a chronic, manageable condition."

The gay community was now looking at an epidemic that had burned through its ranks, killing friends and lovers as well as some of the community's best and brightest, that would not soon be over. Just as the community would continue to grapple, often ineffectively, with the new reality of the AIDS epidemic, the audience that November night failed to grasp the seriousness of the issue they faced.

Reflecting the importance that identities, such as race, gender, and age, and demands for representation had come to play in the community, the single largest category of comments came from those who objected to the membership of the panel.

A sixty-eight-year-old gay man and longtime gay activist rose to point out that only a single panelist had mentioned the elderly in his comments. A black, gay man complained he did not feel he was a part of the gay community that had for so long been dominated by white, gay men. Even one of the two panel members representing youth felt shorted with only two seats on the eight-member panel. There was a single call for unity from a Native American man, a smattering of proposals to deal with the unsafe sex and a call to action from an HIV-positive, gay man. The event left some observers shocked and disappointed.

"I saw a lot of people who were not approaching the problem," said Lou Maletta, at the time the national director of the Gay Cable Network, a producer and distributor of gay news programming in twenty-two American cities.

Spencer Cox, a longtime AIDS activist, said, "Once again there is a group of people in a position to know what they are talking about telling us the sky has fallen. Everybody was too busy being concerned about the ethnic makeup of the panel. It's become clear to me that the community at large has no idea of the bad shape we're in."

If the "community at large" could not comprehend the circumstances that gay men were living under, the community leadership was not doing much better.

In July of 1994, over 150 North American gay and AIDS leaders had gathered in Dallas for a summit "to address the crisis of new infections occurring among gay men, bisexuals, and lesbians at risk for HIV," according to a press release from the American Association of Physicians for Human Rights, a gay doctor's group and the meeting's sponsor.

Carmen Vasquez, a senior staffer at New York City's gay community center, had attended the Dallas summit and she told the audience during the November panel that the conferees had been "overwhelmed by the depth of grief, anger, and despair."

Elovich agreed, saying, "I don't think it's a surprise after the Berlin conference. There's a lot more hopelessness out there in terms of getting a cure."

The summit lasted three days and included multiple plenary sessions, small group discussions, and a day of "intensive discussions." The "proposals for further action," or those items that the community leadership thought were the appropriate responses to this "crisis," were created during the closing session with the proposals generated by inviting the attendees to yell out their suggestions. While that method guaranteed that no views would be censored it also created an unwieldy list. The conferees left Dallas with eighty-nine separate proposals.

Some were ahead of their time in that they called for addressing the role that substance abuse played in HIV transmission, improved HIV surveillance data, or greater coordination between behavioral researchers and those who were implementing HIV prevention programs in the wider community.

Other proposals stated explicitly that they were unrelated to HIV prevention. One called for funding "community-building initiatives" that would "not necessarily be defined as HIV prevention." Another called for combating "bi and transphobia in lesbian and gay organizations," while one sought "deeper discussions involving all genders and sexualities," though the topic of these conversations was not specified. Yet another asked the conferees to "Watch MTV's series *The Real World*, which features young HIV+ gay/bisexual men."

There is a certain irony in one conferee's suggestion that "the needs of gays, lesbians, and bisexuals have to be at the top of the agenda in whatever work we do" because at the close of a three-day conference that was meant "to address the crisis of new infections occurring among gay men, bisexuals, and lesbians at risk for HIV," one attendee proposed that they "brainstorm and create a national gay/lesbian/bisexual prevention campaign." It certainly appeared that the community leadership was not at all sure how to respond to what they described as a "crisis."

Over time, this leadership vacuum would be filled with often rancorous debates concerning the community's approach to HIV prevention, whether oral sex was safe sex, or the role that sex clubs, circuit parties, and bathhouses played in the lives of gay men and the spread of HIV among those men. Just as safe sex was contested when it first appeared, virtually every discussion about gay men's sex lives and safe sex would become an argument. These were often launched by sensational media coverage.

The first of these came in 1992 in New York City after the *Daily News*, a newspaper, *New York* magazine, and a local television news program, which broadcast a two-part series, reported a resurgence in unsafe sex in gay sex clubs, bars, and other businesses.

The broadcast piece featured some footage of sex in a gay bar that was filmed with a hidden camera. The great fallacy in these kinds of broadcast exposés is that they film activity, sex, in this case, that the television stations will not show on the air. Such journalism is unconvincing, but it is also inflammatory and the city was pressed to respond though its response was relatively quiet compared to earlier efforts.

The gay community had seen this sort of coverage before. Roughly seven years earlier, heterosexual hysteria over AIDS had reached its height.

"Around 1984 or 1985 straight people started to realize that AIDS actually existed," Sarah Schulman, the author and activist, said in a 1992 interview with *QW* magazine, a now-defunct gay weekly.

Rock Hudson, the actor, had disclosed his AIDS diagnosis in July of 1985 and died later that year. Health authorities across the nation were discussing closing gay bathhouses and sex clubs. In San Francisco, health authorities closed that city's bathhouses and sex clubs in 1984 with the approval of a local court. The judge who approved the closings called AIDS "a rampant epidemic" and the sex businesses were "a real and present health menace," according to a 1984 story in the *Advocate*. Quarantine as a means of protecting the public health was also debated.

In New York, the state's response, in October of 1985, was to issue a set of "emergency regulations" that banned anal sex and fellatio, with or without a condom, in businesses. The regulations were aimed right at the bathhouses and gay male sex. The regulations would be enforced by local health departments.

The panic, the conspicuous absence of vaginal sex in the regulations, and the general tone of the debate raised, among gay advocates, the very legitimate fear of a wider backlash. In Schulman's 1994 book *My American History*, 1,985 interviews with gay leaders reveal exactly that. Asked if the regulations could lead to an effort to reinstate New York's sodomy laws, which had been struck down by the state's highest court two years before, Virginia Apuzzo, the former executive director of the National Gay Task Force, replied, "That is precisely the link we've been worried about."

In 1992, however, the community response was calmer, in part, because they had not fueled a backlash, but also because the regulations had proved to be relatively toothless. Since they were adopted, the city had only closed eight businesses, including two straight sex clubs, using the regulations.

The wider community was unconcerned. A largely disinterested ACT UP, the radical group that was known for its confrontational tactics, issued a statement calling for community policing of the businesses though the group declined to fulfill that role.

In a 1992 letter, the city's health commissioner, Dr. Margaret A. Hamburg, sought advice from the state AIDS Advisory Council on how to respond to businesses "whose primary function is to provide a public or semi-private space in which patrons may engage in consensual sexual behavior."

The council established a four-person Subcommittee on Sex Clubs that included David Hansell, GMHC's deputy executive director for policy, among its members. The subcommittee, which wanted to "proceed speedily," met just five times and gathered comments from sex club owners, AIDS groups, and a number of other sources.

In a memo distributed to his fellow subcommittee members, Hansell argued that the state regulation should be rewritten to include vaginal sex, to exclude oral sex, and to reflect that where anal or vaginal sex with condoms was happening in a business that should not result in a penalty for that business.

"The encouragement of consistent condom use is a fundamental and widely accepted component of HIV risk reduction education," he wrote. "Not to acknowledge, in an enforcement scheme, the demonstrated value of condoms in preventing HIV transmission would fly in the face of our educational objectives."

Hansell also argued for a regulatory scheme that could include a "fleshed-out 'check-list' of health and safety steps that establishments should implement to encourage safer conduct . . . Furthermore, the city's objective here ought to be putting in place a comprehensive, pro-active risk reduction program that serves sound public health objectives, not a program triggered by sensationalistic media exposes."

The final subcommittee report did not adopt Hansell's views explicitly though it did describe the regulations as "narrow, skewed, and inaccurate" and recommend that they be re-written to "reflect current data about the relative risks of different sexual activities and the distinction between protected (that is, involving the use of a condom) and unprotected activity."

In 1985, the clear intent of the regulations was that they be used to close businesses where gay men were having sex. Some subcommittee members were now effectively suggesting that the state government admit that certain forms of gay and straight sex were valuable and worth preserving. The proposed changes might also have been the start of state regulation of these sex businesses. The state declined to approve anything that resembled regulatory scheme. Only one of the subcommittee's suggestions was given the force of law. The concern that led to the creation of the subcommittee was unsafe sex among gay men and, in early 1993, the state responded by adding vaginal sex to the list of banned behaviors in the state regulations.

The "sensationalistic media exposes" of 1992, however, were mild in comparison to the coverage that came in 1994 and 1995.

Rotello, the author of *Sexual Ecology* and editor of the defunct *Outweek*, a gay magazine, had been hired by *New York Newsday*, a newspaper, as a columnist. In April of 1994, he wrote a column titled, "Sex Clubs Are the Killing Fields of AIDS" in which he described a "sex murder/suicide" that he had witnessed at Zone DK, a New York City sex club that catered to gay men.

"Within minutes of our arrival we happened upon two young men in an open room engaging in unprotected oral sex, the common currency of these clubs," Rotello wrote. "Then, without exchanging a whisper, the two rearranged themselves into the postmodern posture of death: unprotected anal sex, unmistakably without a condom. And in plain view of dozens of their gay male peers."

He critiqued not only the sex club and bathhouse owners, but also AIDS groups that he felt were quick to condemn such things as the American right-wing assaults on safe-sex education, but ignored what might be construed as immoral behavior among gay men.

"But when it comes to challenging the morality of some gay men, especially the culture of promiscuity that some see as the birthright of gay life, suddenly the rhetoric of crisis drops away, replaced with the weak tea of 'education' and 'outreach' and 'condom availability,' or the mock defiant slogan, 'Hands off our clubs,'" he wrote. "If the owners of unsafe sex clubs are like tobacco farmers, the policy wonks at GMHC and the libertarians of ACT UP are like tobacco company spokesmen, all AIDS doublespeak and zero common sense."

Rotello maintained this drumbeat of criticism in additional columns into 1995, but his most stinging charges came in a January 12, 1995, column titled, "Unsafe Sex Clubs: Safe From Crackdowns."

Citing city health department records[3] that showed that agency doing little more than sending form letters to sex businesses threatening them with closure or fines because violations of the state health code were observed in those

3. I obtained these records using the New York State Freedom of Information law and gave them to Rotello and the *Daily News.*

businesses, he mocked the department for its ineffective regulation of the bathhouses and sex clubs. Two weeks later, Rotello wrote, "For Sale: State-of-the-Art Unsafe Sex," a column that described a gay bathhouse that had just opened in Chelsea as "like the legendary bathhouses of old, those bustling hives of contagion that helped spread death throughout the gay male world."

Rotello wrote, "A lot of people, gay and straight, are shocked when they hear that the baths are back. But they shouldn't be. The opening of the West Side Club is a natural development in the context of gay New York's response to the HIV epidemic. We have evolved from almost complete intolerance of commercial multi-partner sex (1986), to muted tolerance as long as it was scrupulously safe (1987–1988), to denial and confusion when it entered the gray zone of possibly unsafe (1989), to indifference when it became blatantly unsafe (1990–today)."

The editorial page of the *Daily News*, which was staffed by Jonathan Capehart, an openly gay journalist, also took up the cause. In an article titled, "Getting Undressed, Going Undercover," he described his experience in the West Side Club.

"My intention was to confirm whether the club is, in fact, the latest representation of a tragic phenomenon: a resurgence in unsafe sex among gays," he wrote. "I discovered, with almost complete certitude, that the answer is yes."

A group of gay men, including Rotello, formed the Gay and Lesbian HIV Prevention Activists[4] to advocate for stricter city controls on sex clubs and bathhouses.

Among the GALPHA supporters was Michelangelo Signorile, author of *Life Outside: The Signorile Report on Sex, Drugs,*

4. I was a GALHPA member.

Muscles, and the Passages of Life, an ACT UP member, a former *Outweek* contributor, and a columnist with *Out,* joined the fray with columns in *Out.* With his usual aggressive style, Signo-rile fired directly at those he was debating.

"Some people, small in number but quite vocal and pow-erful (including some of those charged with developing HIV prevention strategies in our AIDS organizations), put politics above sound prevention, fearful that making further sacrifices when it comes to sexual behavior—even in the midst of an epidemic—amounts to ceding sexual freedom to the right wing," he wrote in late 1995.

For the GALHPA members, the gay community was pre-sented with a crisis that required a quick and dramatic response. In a 1995 editorial published in the *Daily News,* Andrew M. Beaver, a GALHPA founder, wrote that they had called on AIDS groups, including GMHC, to respond to reports of increased unsafe sex a year earlier and had been rebuffed. AIDS, in their view, was a far greater threat to the community than a theoretical concern over rights.

"To put civil libertarian ideology ahead of common-sense efforts to reduce HIV transmission is wrong," Beaver wrote. "As gay men we must be willing to recognize that ending the AIDS epidemic will not come without sacrifice. Allowing the city to close unsafe sex clubs is not a dangerous infringement of our rights. It is but a small price to pay so that our com-munity may live."

Two GALHPA members[5] took Amy Pagnozzi, a *Daily News* columnist, disguised with a fake moustache, into Zone DK in a failed effort to expose the unsafe sex in the club. Pagnozzi, who observed no unsafe sex there, noted that as a

5. I was one of the two.

result of the recent press coverage the sex club had "cleaned up its act."

The *Daily News* editorial page went on to cite the same health department letters that Rotello had discussed and demand that the city "shut sex clubs now." The paper printed additional editorials demanding action. That proved to be too much for Mayor Rudolph W. Giuliani, a Republican who had just started his first term in 1994. When GALHPA demanded a meeting with City Hall, they quickly got it.

The March meeting[6] drew Peter Powers, the first deputy mayor, essentially the city's second-in-command, Hamburg, the health commissioner, Ronald Johnson, the city's AIDS czar, Wilfredo Lopez, the health department's general counsel, and a number of other city officials. GALHPA presented the city with eight demands that were intended "To end HIV transmission in commercial sex establishments" and included the requirement that all spaces in city sex businesses must be "monitorable." That meant that the doors on private rooms in the city's bathhouses had to come off. The owners must be required to hire monitors and to deliver safe-sex education and tools, such as lube and condoms, to their customers, GALHPA said.

Recognizing that it was unlikely that the state health code was going to be revised, GALHPA simply stated, among its eight points, "Sexual activity on the premises must comply with health-code regulations."

As the March meeting ended, Lopez turned to a GALHPA member and said, incredulously, "You want us to regulate these businesses?" "Yes," was the answer. The city responded just as the state had responded two years earlier. At a second March meeting, this time with Hamburg, Johnson, and a

6. I attended this meeting.

special assistant to Powers, GALHPA was told that the city was "very sympathetic," but that incorporating its eight points into the city code "would not be appropriate." GALHPA's proposals were dead on arrival, but the city did begin aggressively enforcing the state health code.

In 1995, the health department made between thirteen hundred and fourteen hundred separate inspections of between forty and fifty businesses. Thirty received warning letters and, at least, nine were closed. In 1996, the health department sent warning letters to eleven businesses and closed, at least, eleven clubs. The city warned one business and temporarily closed another in 1997. In 1998 and 1999, a task force of inspectors from the police, fire, health, and buildings departments, under the auspices of the Mayor's Office of Midtown Enforcement, made multiple inspections of the city's bathhouses. The city closed one bathhouse in 1999.

The Giuliani administration took full advantage of the controversy that GALHPA had created. Other New Yorkers who were less concerned with unsafe sex among gay men and more concerned about property values had been complaining about the growth of porn shops and theaters across the city. Additionally, both the city and New York State had long wanted to remove the porn shops and theaters that had proliferated in New York City's midtown and replace them with businesses that were more tourist-friendly.

In 1995, the city enacted zoning legislation that sharply limited where such businesses could operate. While the city was pursuing these porn shops using the zoning regulations and, in some cases, the state was seizing them under eminent domain laws, roughly 70 percent of the businesses that were closed for violating the state health code were also businesses that were subject to the porn shop zoning law.

Although the Giuliani administration might have discovered that it could use the state health regulations to close porn shops on its own, it certainly appears that GALHPA handed City Hall a weapon and the GALHPA members soon found themselves scrambling to put distance between their agenda and Giuliani's.

In the gay community, GALHPA was attacked. While Rotello's earlier columns had drawn some angry rebukes, the gay community opposition to GALHPA's proposals was widespread and heated.

A mere twenty-five people had signed GALHPA's original statement that announced its eight-point plan. At a town meeting[7] held at New York City's gay community center the week before GALHPA met with city officials, several hundred people gathered and it was clear from audience or panelist comments, or the applause those comments drew, that they objected strongly to GALHPA's plan.

In a March 1995 *Village Voice* article that detailed the debate, Gregg Gonsalves, a longtime gay and AIDS activist, called the GALHPA members "rogue activists." Another such activist, Stephen Gendin, described the GALHPA proposals as "calling on the police to watch over us" in the *Village Voice* article. Gay men were simply not going to support anything that resembled government regulation of their sex lives.

In June of 1995, thirty leading gay or AIDS groups and individuals wrote the Giuliani administration to express their opposition to the GALHPA proposals. The signatories included GMHC, the gay community center, the Empire State Pride Agenda, the statewide gay lobbying group, ACT UP, the Lambda Legal Defense and Education Fund, a gay

7. Rotello and I represented GALHPA on the panel at this meeting.

law group, and the New York City Gay and Lesbian Anti-Violence Project.

"As leaders in the lesbian and gay community and in the fight against AIDS, we support AIDS prevention," the letter read. "But not every measure proposed in the name of prevention is consistent with that goal. The state health-code regulation of commercial sex establishments, for example, contradicts the consensus of public health experts . . . [The measure fails] to distinguish between protected and unprotected sex. [It treats] as equivalent a range of sex acts—oral, anal and vaginal intercourse—that have widely different degrees of risk."

Some of the people who attended the town meeting formed the AIDS Prevention Action League, which sought and won its own meeting with the city. The group asked that the city not enforce the health code and instead allow the community to police the sex clubs. The city rejected that request.

APAL also published their own editorials in the mainstream press, produced its own safe sex materials, held its own sex parties, and worked with one New York City sex club to try and implement safe-sex practices there. "We want to see if it's possible to transform a club," said Gendin, an APAL founder, who died in 2000.

For APAL and Sex Panic!, the group that eventually replaced APAL, the debate concerned more than just fighting the state health code and GALHPA's plan. They were opposing what they saw as government regulation of gay men's bodies.

In a 1995 interview on National Public Radio, Gendin said that the failure of HIV prevention was recent and it was "way too early to start going to the government, especially a government that's becoming increasingly conservative and that increasingly has its own agenda of limiting sexuality and sort of shutting down gay places anyway."

They were also asserting that there was value in the sex that gay men were having in these businesses. In the same NPR piece, historian Allan Berube, the author of *Coming Out Under Fire: The History of Gay Men and Women in World War II*, said, "For me, it's the adventure of meeting someone you don't know and feeling this erotic charge and, you know, exploring them and their bodies and having conversations and having this kind of bond with someone that you never met before and may never meet again. There's this specialness about that kind of intimacy with a stranger, that there's nothing else like it and it's its own thing."

Within six months, GALHPA had stopped meeting and the group's work was effectively finished, but the controversy that its proposals spawned persisted. That debate continued in the *Advocate* and *Out, Newsday, the Daily News, Lesbian and Gay New York* and other mainstream and gay publications into 1996 and 1997.

Rotello's *Sexual Ecology* and Signorile's *Life Outside* were also published in 1997. Both books explored how the sexual culture that gay men had built made the epidemic possible and kept it growing. Those messages made both authors targets of the gay left. Despite their radical credentials, both were vilified as reactionaries and, in a charge that is seen as particularly damning in some gay circles, sex negative.

Sex Panic!, a group that included some of the gay and lesbian community's leading thinkers and activists, emerged as the dominant influence in the debate, according to a 1997 article in *Lingua Franca*, a now defunct journal of academia.

Among its members were Michael Warner, a Rutgers University professor, author of *The Trouble with Normal: Sex, Politics, and the Ethics of Queer Life*, and "one of the deans of queer theory," according to *Lingua Franca*. The Sex Panic! roster also included Douglas Crimp, whose essay, "How to Have Promiscuity in a Epidemic," published in the journal *October* in 1987, recalled the 1983 Callen/Berkowitz safe-sex pamphlet, and Kendall Thomas, a professor at Columbia University's law school.

"It's a Who's Who of queer theory," said one graduate student in the *Lingua Franca* piece. These leading queer theorists "realized that the state regulation of public sex was an activity they wanted to oppose," the journal reported.

Sex Panic!, which eventually had chapters in several other American cities, including San Francisco and San Diego, was defending against what it saw as attacks on gay sexuality. One Sex Panic! flyer, that invited the public to a teach-in, featured the text, "Danger! Assault! Turdz."

The danger was that "HIV continues to spread. A new generation is at risk. Meanwhile we feel burnout and despair. Sexual liberation is mocked."

The assault came from a government that was imposing the porn shop zoning regulations, arresting gay men for having sex in public, and shuttering sex businesses frequented by those men.

"Queer New York is being shut down. Not since Stonewall have we faced so much harassment," the flyer read. The "Turdz" were Andrew Sullivan, Signorile, Larry Kramer, and Rotello.

"They say we caused AIDS: they blame us for spreading it: they tell us to get married . . . they don't like gay culture, they don't believe in safer sex, they don't trust you," the flyer read. Sex Panic! was the latest defender of sexual liberation though its defense had a distinctly different tone.

"The phenomenology of a sex club encounter is an experience of world making," Warner told *Lingua Franca*. "It's an experience of being connected not just to this person but to potentially limitless numbers of people, and that's why it's important that it be with a stranger. Sex with a stranger is like a metonym."

As the health department's enforcement of the state health code faded in 1997 and the porn shops and theaters mounted an aggressive legal response to the porn shop zoning law, Sex Panic! was increasingly without a cause. Noting that the sex club business seemed to thriving in New York City and any city crackdown had ended, the *Lingua Franca* story asked, "If Sex Panic! has not been crying wolf, its members need to explain why."

Yet another debate had ended with a whimper and the gay community no closer to addressing the crisis that all the players claimed motivated them. Many of the participants in the debate over sex clubs and bathhouses were also battling over the relative safety of oral sex.

In 1994, Rotello published a long story in *Out* magazine titled, "Watch Your Mouth: The Word Is in on HIV and Oral Sex and It Isn't Good" that warned that the risk of acquiring HIV through oral sex might be higher than many gay men and AIDS groups had assumed.

There had been case reports of both men and women becoming infected with HIV through oral sex dating back to 1984, but studies that attempted to define the risk of infection through oral sex typically found that it was not a risk factor. Among gay men and the AIDS groups that serve them, oral sex was generally assumed to be low risk and, for many AIDS groups, that risk was low enough that they promoted oral sex as a safe alternative to anal sex.

Rotello was challenging the consensus. He cited the stories of gay men who believed they had been infected through oral sex. He relied on a 1993 San Francisco study that found cases of HIV transmission through oral sex and concluded that the risk of such infections was higher than previously known. He made the same point in a 1995 column in *Newsday* column titled, "The Ominous Odds of Unprotected Sex."

Rotello also noted a flaw in the study of the relative risks of oral sex versus anal sex. In most studies, when an HIV-positive gay man said he had engaged in both types of sex the cause of his infection was inevitably assigned to the anal sex so the contribution of oral sex to the spread of HIV was masked.

Among those who sparred with Rotello was Odets who charged in a 1995 *Harper's* article and in a two-part piece in the *San Francisco Sentinel* that Rotello was misrepresenting data and he defended the prevailing view that oral sex was low risk.

"Fortunately, there is a well-kept, often misrepresented secret in America about the data on oral sex: Virtually all research suggests that under ordinary circumstances oral sex is an extremely low risk activity for transmitting HIV," he wrote in the *Sentinel*.

The strongest defense of oral sex came during the eleventh International Conference on AIDS, held in Vancouver in 1968,[8] when GMHC organized what was a "standing-room-only forum" on oral sex, according to a 1996 *Village Voice* article.

That same year, GMHC published a pamphlet on oral sex titled, "To Suck or Not to Suck: Only You Can Decide What You Put in Your Mouth" that concluded that oral sex is "low risk." The forum had clearly been organized to affirm that conclusion.

---

8. After the tenth conference in 1994, the event began meeting every other year.

The *Village Voice* reported that after hearing from three researchers who said that "although some people have been infected through oral sex, such cases appear to be rare."

One of the researchers, Dr. David G. Ostrow, who was affiliated with Chicago's Howard Brown Health Center, argued for preserving oral sex using language that was similar to that used by Sex Panic! in the bathhouse debate. Oral sex has "a value and meaning that could outweigh the risks," he told the *Village Voice* and to deny that is "sex-negative."

The forum ended with comments from Eric Rofes, a long-time gay and AIDS activist and the author of, among other books, *Reviving the Tribe: Regenerating Gay Men's Sexuality and Culture in the Ongoing Epidemic*, published in 1996, and *Dry Bones Breathe: Gay Men Creating Post-AIDS Identities and Cultures*, published in 1998.

"'The oral sex panic,' he declared, arises from 'a deeply rooted anxiety about what we do with our bodies with other males' and from society's dismissal of 'the authentic need that many men have to exchange semen,'" the *Village Voice* reported. Rofes concluded by telling the audience to "hold our ground" on oral sex and, "If you want to make it even more safe, don't let him come in your mouth. But keep doing it," according to the *Village Voice*.

At the same conference, however, one researcher presented data on twelve cases of new HIV infections. In four of those cases, oral sex was identified as the cause. The researcher told the *Village Voice* that "oral transmission of HIV may occur more often than previously recognized" and "if you perform oral sex enough times, your cumulative risk could be substantial." The *Village Voice* noted other studies that found similar numbers.

That same year, the Gay and Lesbian Medical Association, previously known as the American Association of Physicians for Human Rights, released a study that also concluded that oral sex was "low risk."

When it came to oral sex, gay men were left to fend for themselves. It was generally low risk, but, as some studies noted, under certain circumstances that risk could change.

The bathhouse and oral sex debates revealed the difficult position that gay and AIDS groups occupied in these disputes. Even if they had supported GALHPA's positions, and none did, or believed that HIV prevention efforts should reflect the view that oral sex might carry a higher risk of HIV transmission than previously known, and some leading AIDS activists believed that, they would risk offending the community they served, their staff, volunteers, and donors, many of whom were gay, if they endorsed the radical changes proposed by GALHPA or voiced a new view of oral sex. In the debate over circuit parties, however, these AIDS agencies were at the center of the dispute.

The controversy began in earnest in 1996 when a gay man overdosed, apparently on GHB, at the fourteenth annual Morning Party, a GMHC fund-raiser held on the beach, usually in August, in the Pines section of Fire Island. The man, who recovered, was flown by helicopter to a Long Island hospital. The party had been criticized for the drug use there by Andrew Sullivan in the *New Republic* in 1993 and concerns about drug use at the event were raised in a 1995 article in *New York* magazine.

Days prior to the 1996 party, a letter, on GMHC stationery and apparently sent from the agency's executive director and board, was distributed to the residents of the Pines. The authors of the hoax letter wrote that GMHC could no longer participate in the Morning Party because of the "widespread drug use" at the event that "often leads to unsafe sex."

The *New York Times* covered the hoax letter and the controversy in an article that appeared the day before the party. The critics included Larry Kramer, the playwright and a GMHC founder, and Adam R. Rose, a real estate executive who was described as a "former donor" to GMHC.

"A party whose point is really drug use has no place benefiting an organization that is fighting for intelligent decisions that lead to safer sex," Rose told the *Times*. Kramer said of the drug use, "We started the organization to change all that, not perpetuate it." He added that he had attended the Morning Party two years earlier and "I was pretty shocked . . . It was as if AIDS had never happened and I was back in 1974 again. The drugs were rampant and so was the sexuality of it all, the hedonism. I was ashamed of GMHC's affiliation with it."

Party sponsors, gay men, and other gay community leaders defended GMHC and noted that the party included efforts to educate attendees about drug use.

"It successfully engages many people who might not otherwise be engaged in this battle," Richard D. Burns, executive director of the gay community center, told the *Times*. "The Morning Party is a successful celebration in Fire Island of a community that has a long history and association with GMHC."

GMHC then distributed its own response in which it reaffirmed its support for the party. "In reality, GMHC is proud to continue its longest-running fund-raising event," the agency wrote. If the 1996 Morning Party had been a piece of theater, the overdose could not have been more perfectly timed.

The major daily newspapers in New York all took note of the overdose and the *Daily News* editorial page, with a piece titled "Gay Group's Ethical Hangover," took GMHC to task for its involvement with the party.

"Gay Men's Health Crisis has a dirty little secret that is finally getting out," the piece read. "The annual Fire Island fund-raiser for the nation's premiere AIDS services organization has become a drug fest, rampant with the kind of destructive behavior the group was formed to fight."

Michael T. Isbell, GMHC's associate executive director, answered the editorial forcefully in a letter to the editor.

"Open your eyes, *Daily News*," he wrote. "It's no 'dirty little secret' that drug and alcohol use exist at gay parties like the Morning Party . . . Nor is it a secret that shaming people who drink and use drugs, or calling the behavior dirty, doesn't really fix the problem—gay men have been called dirty and shameful for years. GMHC doesn't serve drugs, we don't promote drugs, and no, we don't search or interrogate the adults who go to our events. We do have free, nationally recognized counseling and education programs that talk honestly about substance abuse rather than wishing it all away."

The *Daily News* responded with a column from Capehart who wrote that the Isbell letter "must have come from GMHC's department of cheap shots. But the real shame is Isbell's refusal to answer the question: Does GMHC realize that its sponsorship of the drug-soaked Morning Party and it noble history of being 'first in the fight against AIDS' do not mix?"

The controversy returned the next year when the *Times* published an editorial by Michelangelo Signorile, the day before the 1997 party took place, that criticized GMHC and expanded the debate by noting that other AIDS organizations were also receiving funds from circuit parties.

"AIDS groups, like other charities, are always looking for new ways to raise money, and they began tapping into the party circuit almost since its inception," he wrote. "But this relationship has been troubled from the start, and is only becoming more so. There is something hypocritical about groups that try to encourage healthful lifestyles, but that benefit from parties where drugs have become a problem, even if the sponsoring groups have worked to address drug abuse."

In a follow-up story a week later the *Times* noted that there had been twenty-one arrests for drug possession at the 1997 party. The article also noted that the controversy that attached to the party continued.

In 1998, there were also twenty-one drug possession arrests, but more significantly, several hours before the party began a New York man died from a GHB overdose and three friends of his were hospitalized after taking the drug. While none of the press coverage asserted that the four men were on Fire Island to attend the party, the death became associated with the Morning Party and, in early 1999, GMHC announced it would no longer produce the event.

Beginning in 1997, the relationships between circuit parties and other AIDS groups were explored in the mainstream and gay press. The coverage noted the continued drug problems and overdoses at the events. While some groups defended their choice to take cash from the parties, others pointedly noted that they refused circuit party funds.

"I think there is an epidemic of sexual addiction and drug addiction, and the circuit is where those two paths cross," said Michael Weinstein, president of the Los Angeles AIDS Healthcare Foundation, who told the *Los Angeles Times* in 1997 that his organization did not take money from a local circuit party.

By 2001, the *Southern Voice*, a gay newspaper published in Atlanta, wrote that some AIDS groups in that city had rejected funds from one circuit party produced there.

"There was a lot of controversy a number of years ago

regarding unsafe behavior at circuit parties," Stephen Woods, executive director of Project Open Hand, an AIDS group that delivers meals to people living with terminal diseases, told the newspaper.

These debates were not the only issues that drew the attention of the gay community. Barebacking, or intentional unprotected anal sex, and to a lesser extent "bug chasing," or seeking to become infected, and "gift giving," or seeking to infect another, all made an appearance.

The earliest reference to barebacking, though he did not call it that, came in an editorial titled "Exit the Rubberman" by Scott O'Hara, publisher and editor of *Steam*, a "quarterly journal for men," in a 1995 issue. O'Hara, who died in 1998, was HIV-positive and declared that "I'm tired of using condoms and I won't." Like many of the early barebackers, O'Hara also said he would not have sex with men who were uninfected.

"The essence of fucking, to me, is not penetration per se, but trust: I trust you to be gentle (or rough, or whatever), I trust you to make me feel good, I trust you enough to want your cum up my ass," he wrote. "Wearing a condom negates those feelings ... I want a man, but not a Negative any longer, not a man who's scared of the juices of my body. The Negative world is defined by fear, ours by pleasure, and it takes another Positive to treat me with the abandon for which sex was invented."

Roughly two years later, in June of 1997, Gendin, the APAL founder, expressed similar views in a *Poz* article titled "Riding Bareback: Skin-On-Skin Sex Been There, Done That, Want More." For Gendin, bareback sex had a powerful emotional appeal.

"When he came inside me, I was in heaven, just overjoyed," he wrote. "Knowing the guy was positive made it empowering, not guilt-inspiring. I relaxed into my desires instead of fighting them and felt good doing so . . . I can't comment on a negative guy's decision to go raw, but for us positive men, the benefits are obvious. The physical sensation is much better. The connection feels closer and more intimate."

The mainstream press took note of barebacking in a September 1997 *Newsweek* story titled "A Deadly Dance." The story also mentioned "gift giving" and "bug chasing" though, like all stories on these two phenomena, it provided scant evidence of their existence.

The controversy over barebacking came to a head in November of 1997 at Creating Change, an annual conference organized by the National Gay and Lesbian Task Force, when Tony Valenzuela, a twenty-nine-year-old, HIV-positive, gay man addressed a town meeting there.

After publishing a six-part series titled, "Sex Panic!" in *Gay and Lesbian Times*, a newspaper in San Diego, Valenzuela had assisted in organizing a day-long Sex Panic! summit that took place in San Diego at the same time as Creating Change. The town meeting was a Creating Change panel discussion and it only included Sex Panic! members and supporters, such as Eric Rofes.

What had been, for O'Hara and Gendin, a personal declaration of the allure of unprotected sex became, for Valenzuela, a political statement and an indictment of HIV prevention efforts. He stunned some in the crowd of 2,000 who attended the event when he discussed his unprotected sex.

"I am a sex radical," he said, according to the text of his speech that was reprinted in *Gay Community News*, a Boston quarterly. "I have always been highly sexual, promiscuous, adventurous, and creative with my sexual appetite. I am a sex gourmet in a community serving sexual TV dinners."

Valenzuela laid the responsibility for his infection on failed
HIV prevention messages and said, "I've moved away from
looking for HIV prevention solutions, I've placed myself in
the middle of HIV anarchy, there trying to understand risk
and desire, the pleasure of barebacking and cum, the interest
I hold in promiscuity . . . While immersing myself in HIV
anarchy I've concluded one thing: HIV prevention alone will
never contain this virus. I strongly believe, for a significant
portion of gay men, no prevention message will ever work and
so therefore there will always be seroconversions."

In some parts of the gay and lesbian community Valenzuela
was attacked for his comments. Barebacking was seen as the
latest threat to stemming new HIV infections among gay
men. Valenzuela and Sex Panic! were charged with being proponents of unsafe sex.

"Most frightening about Valenzuela's speech was that a
small group of mostly middle-aged gay leftist men, known as
Sex Panic!, are using him as their poster boy," Rich Tafel,
executive director of the Log Cabin Republicans, a gay
group, wrote in a 1998 editorial that was published in the *San
Francisco Chronicle*. "These men pretend that the gay community hasn't been decimated by AIDS, using the language
of freedom and individual rights to justify sexual behavior
that can be deadly . . . But today, with all of the risks known,
Sex Panic! romanticizes being HIV-positive, almost
implying to young people that if you aren't positive, you're
not fully gay."

Valenzuela also had his defenders. In a 1999 *Poz* profile of
Valenzuela—the cover story on him featured a photo of him
lying naked on the back of a horse—Rofes praised Valenzuela
for telling the truth.

"By discussing anal sex as a valuable, meaningful act for

many gay men, Valenzuela shattered a powerful taboo that had taken root during the crisis years of the AIDS epidemic," Rofes said. "We'd become accustomed to expecting fags to maintain a public silence about the wide discrepancy between the ways many AIDS groups publicly represented gay men's sex lives, and what we knew was occurring in gay communities throughout the nation."

Valenzuela made the same argument in a 1999 town meeting on barebacking held in New York City. While his rhetoric had cooled since 1997, he told the crowd of roughly 200 people, "It isn't just that I told the truth. It's much more than that. I also offered a critique of HIV prevention."

The same *Poz* issue that featured Valenzuela on the cover also included a story by writer Michael Scarce that discussed barebacking as an emerging political movement and noted that the barebackers were organizing through the Internet.

"The controversy continues with a growing recognition that barebacking is neither a fad nor a glamorous buzzword," Scarce wrote. "It remains to be seen how politicized barebackers will become about their rights and responsibilities. While it's unlikely that a contingent of bareback advocates will march in this year's gay pride parades, this community is increasingly visible."

Speaking at the 1999 town meeting, Scarce said, "I'm talking about men who have made a really firm decision to not use condoms. It's kind of this grassroots thing that is out there . . . It clearly has a great deal of value and intrinsic meaning to these men's lives . . . Barebackers are being politicized and they are doing organizing around condomless sex."

At that same meeting, GMHC's Elovich dismissed the *Poz* cover as "marketing" and added that "explicit or provocative is not always informative." He observed that the barebacking credo, or "waving the flag of barebacking pride," was mere sloganeering that was little different from what he termed the "catechism" of safe sex. A gay man can say he will use a condom every time, but "with certain circumstances and certain people maybe you'll change your mind," Elovich said.

"We need to help men gain pleasure and control over their bodies," Elovich said. "Simpleminded messages or dogma just doesn't cut it anymore."

Even those who had been inclined to express some support for Valenzuela two years earlier appeared to be less sympathetic in 1999.

"All I hear is a critique of prevention, but I don't hear the prevention," said Warner of Sex Panic! at the town meeting. "What do you intend on doing, not for barebackers, but for all the people in the penumbra around it."

Scarce, like *Newsweek* before him, noted the appearance of bug chasers and gift givers in his *Poz* story.

"Rare exceptions to the barebacking norm, these men prize not just unprotected anal sex or even semen but HIV itself as the ultimate intimacy to share with another," Scarce wrote in a piece titled, "A Ride on the Wild Side." "In a mind-boggling feat of symbolic reversal, they have taken the dread and deadliness of the virus and transformed it into desire and regeneration."

Bug chasing and gift giving would reappear in a 2003 in a highly controversial *Rolling Stone* article that was criticized for its complete absence of any gift givers, just a few bug chasers, and a glaring error in its estimate of the number of HIV infections that might be attributed to these two activities. Other 2003 stories on these topics in the mainstream press were notable for their lack of gift givers and bug chasers, often quoted anonymously, who seemed to be having an impossible time finding someone to infect them with HIV.

In 1999, Elovich summed up what is to this day the prevailing view among researchers and HIV prevention activists on bug chasing and gift giving.

"It is ridiculous to suggest that there is a wave of bug chasers out there actively seeking infection and powering the epidemic," he said.

Barebacking, "bug chasing," and "gift giving" were not the only panics that seized the attention of the press. African-American gay and bisexual men had a moment in the media spotlight.

In 2003, the *New York Times Magazine*, the *Washington Post*, and the *Chicago Sun-Times* published stories saying that men on the "down low," or African-American men who have sex with both men and women, but do not identify as gay or bisexual, were making a significant contribution to the spread of HIV among African-Americans.

Each story cited data from the Young Men's Survey, a multi-year, multi-city study by Dr. Linda A. Valleroy, a CDC researcher, to assert that these men were a bridge for HIV from the gay community to heterosexuals. The Chicago and New York papers also relied on testimony from J. L. King, an African-American man who wrote a book about his experience on the "down low." Very quickly, the standard representation of these men in popular culture became that they were dishonest men who threatened the health of African-American women. What was missing was any data to support that assertion.

The CDC grew sufficiently concerned about how its Young Men's Survey data was being used that, in a 2004 press release that accompanied new data from the survey, it pointedly noted that the study was not about down low or bisexual men.

"YMS was not a 'down low sample of young men,' YMS was not a 'bisexual sample of young men,'" she wrote in an e-mail to *Gay City News*. "YMS was a sample of young men who had ever had sex with men who went to venues where young men who had sex with men were likely to go. The reason that 'down-low' appears in the press release from CDC is that CDC was afraid that the press would get the wrong idea: the wrong idea being that YMS studied down low or bisexual guys, solely or particularly."

By the start of the twenty-first century, it seemed that the gay community could not get beyond a cycle of inflammatory press coverage spawning a debate or intense attention to an issue only to have interest in these matters fade quickly.

As these debates and panics were taking place, the appearance of powerful, new anti-HIV drugs prompted some in the gay male community and the mainstream press to suggest that AIDS either had been, or was about to be, defeated. The view that the fight against AIDS was close to finished led others to argue for an approach to gay men's health that included HIV as one of a number of concerns. Chief among those who argued that the AIDS epidemic had ended was Andrew Sullivan, the commentator and author of *Virtually Normal: An Argument About Homosexuality*.

In "When Plagues End: Notes on the Twilight of an Epidemic," a 1996 article that ran in the *New York Times Magazine*, Sullivan observed that the powerful new anti-HIV drugs had dramatically changed the nature of AIDS. That observation was entirely accurate. Those drugs had saved the lives of thousands of gay men, including Sullivan's, though he recognized that this was not a universal experience. Others, including some who were far more knowledgeable about AIDS than Sullivan, did not share his view that these drugs represented the end of the epidemic.

"Most official statements about AIDS—the statements by responsible scientists, by advocate organizations, by doctors— do not, of course, concede that this plague is over," Sullivan wrote. "And, in one sense, obviously, it is not. Someone today will be infected with HIV. The vast majority of HIV-positive people in the world, and a significant minority in America, will not have access to the expensive and effective new drug treatments now available. And many Americans—especially blacks and Latinos—will still die. Nothing I am saying here is meant to deny that fact, or to mitigate its awfulness."

Still, the new drugs mean that "a diagnosis of HIV infection is not just different in degree today than, say, five years ago. It is different in kind. It no longer signifies death. It merely signifies illness," Sullivan wrote.

The major weekly news magazines joined the chorus in 1996. *Time* named Dr. David D. Ho, head of the Aaron Diamond AIDS Research Center, its Man of the Year for his theory that early and aggressive treatment of HIV, or "hit early, hit hard" as it was called, might eradicate the virus in the body. That practice has since been abandoned. In a cover story, *Newsweek* asked "The End of AIDS? Not Yet—But New Drugs Offer Hope."

Publishing in the *Village Voice* in 1997, Dan Savage, the sex advice guru, announced that "The AIDS Crisis Is Over—For Me." Savage wrote that the anti-HIV drugs meant that for one group of Americans, the middle class, HIV was no longer a death sentence. He also observed that he and his partner, both were HIV-negative, had given up using condoms before they confirmed their HIV status because they believed that the drugs were effective treatments. Savage published additional articles on these themes in *The Stranger*, a Seattle alternative weekly newspaper.

In *Dry Bones Breathe*, Rofes argued that the gay community had encountered its "protease moment," a reference to one class of anti-HIV drugs, when "all social and cultural changes in our experiences of the AIDS epidemic were explained in light of the new therapies." Rofes correctly noted that the new drugs had fundamentally changed how gay men perceived HIV and AIDS. The terror that gay men experienced in the 1980s was gone. He faulted AIDS groups for not responding to this.

"That raises an issue prevention leaders seem unable to confront, which ultimately may make or break prevention organizations in the coming years," he wrote. "In epicenter cities since 1995, while many remain infected with HIV, significantly fewer gay men are sick and dying than in the 1990s. We expect men either not to notice this shift in the material reality of their lives, or to allow it to have no effect on their worldviews and the ways they organize their erotic lives."

Rofes also wrote that, generally, the "protease moment" required AIDS groups to restructure their programs to include HIV prevention efforts as part of a broader effort addressing gay men's health.

"It may be appropriate for some gay groups to keep HIV prevention in a prominent position in their mission statements and in their organizational work," he wrote. "Yet I believe that maintaining a narrow focus on reducing infections, as opposed to placing this aim in a context of general overall health promotion, triggers a single-mindedness that easily shifts into moralizing and subtle coercion."

Rofes was also a leader in the gay men's health movement that organized three national meetings, in 1999, 2000, and

2003, and spawned a series of similar regional meetings that sought to expand the health concerns in gay men's lives beyond AIDS. Topics at the summits included aging, drug use, spirituality, and a range of other matters.

"From 1983 to 1993, gay men experienced AIDS as a crisis," Rofes told the *Denver Post* during the 2000 event. "But I'm not sure you can experience it as a crisis for more than ten years . . Now it's time to look at AIDS and gay men's health more holistically."

At the 2003 summit, held in North Carolina, HIV prevention had gone from being one health concern among many to something that may be threatening the health of gay men. In an interview with the *Durham Herald Sun*, Rofes said, "The way I would put it is an AIDS-centric approach to working with gay men may be the problem rather than the solution. When you consistently approach a stigmatized population with concern about one specific health issue and one specific virus, it on some level encourages them to be less concerned about other challenges. So, for example, if you raise a population of young gay men with the repeated idea that AIDS is the end of the world and it's what's going to get them, how dangerous do they consider other things like syphilis, like substance abuse, like violence?"

The views championed by Sullivan, Savage, Rofes and the mainstream press were disputed in the gay and mainstream press with some charging that they were painting a far too rosy picture of the state of the epidemic.

In a 1997 editorial that was published widely in the gay press, Dr. John D'Emilio, a historian and a director at the National Gay and Lesbian Task Force, challenged the mainstream press view in "The End of AIDS? Not Exactly."

While stating that the drop in AIDS deaths was "very

hopeful news," D'Emilio wrote that "the view that the end of AIDS is in sight" is "as dangerous as it is wrongheaded and unwarranted."

D'Emilio wrote that there was much that was unknown about the drugs. Who would pay for them? How long would they be effective? Will those taking the drugs develop drug-resistant HIV?

"I don't want to pour water on the hopefulness that some good news engenders," D'Emilio wrote. "But we need to be very clear about what the end of AIDS would really look like: no more deaths from AIDS, and a prevention effort that leads to an absence of new infections. We are not there yet, and we will only get there through the implementation of policies that require political courage: needle exchange; prevention campaigns that speak frankly about sexual behavior; a level of funding that will accelerate medical breakthroughs; and a national commitment to health care access for everyone."

In a piece that recalled Larry Kramer's 1983 *Village Voice* article "2,339 and Counting," the number referred to the AIDS cases diagnosed to date, Signorile took Rofes, Sullivan and Savage to task in a piece titled "641,086 and Counting" in Out in 1998. Signorile predicted a "disaster" brought on, in part, by the drugs and, in part, by the "hype" surrounding the drugs.

"A disaster in which safer-sex practices among gay men continue to diminish, in part due to that hype, as many gay men blindly believe the drugs make AIDS 'manageable' and that it's not so bad to get HIV," he wrote. "A disaster in which drug-resistant strains of HIV—mutations of the virus bred in the bodies of some people with HIV in response to the drug therapy—begin spreading rapidly. A disaster in which our now-downsized AIDS-service organizations, as well as private and public health-care facilities that have cut back services because their AIDS caseloads dropped, become overwhelmed with very sick people."

Perhaps the loudest voice declaring the end of AIDS came in 1999 when the *New York Times* published a story describing a survey of 7,650 gay and bisexual men done by GMHC and New York City's health department. The story, titled "New York Study Finds Gay Men Using Safer Sex," appeared on page one, above the fold, the day after New York City's Gay Pride March when many in the community rush to a nearby newsstand to check the coverage of the prior day's march.

Citing the survey, the *Times* reported that "HIV infection rates among gay men are lower than commonly believed" and "that young gay men are heeding messages about the need for precautions, contrary to fears that unprotected sex has been increasing." The story was one of largely unqualified success.

"It shows that prevention is working," Dr. Tracy J. Mayne, a health department epidemiologist told the *Times*. "HIV prevalence is decreasing in New York City, no question. We have cut the rate at least in half."

The Associated Press and *Newsday* provided more skeptical coverage, but the *Times*'s influence is such that these stories had little impact. Critics of the survey remained silent.

In one respect, the *Times*, Rofes, and others were correct. Just as they had done in the 1980s, a portion of gay men, perhaps even the majority, had taken steps to protect themselves or reduce their risk of becoming infected. Their critics often failed to take note of these men.

What Rofes, the *Times*, and others failed to take note of was what the Lingua Franca article called the "stubborn remainder" who continued to be unsafe and might have been emboldened by the new drugs to have even more unsafe sex. These were the men that Signorile had discussed in his 1998 article.

By the mid-1990s, AIDS groups were confronting the "stubborn remainder" and they understood that drug and alcohol use played a large role in the unsafe sex among these men. Notwithstanding Rofes's characterization of AIDS groups potentially lapsing into "moralizing and subtle coercion," most of the groups that served gay men were headed in the opposite direction and adopting harm reduction as the organizing philosophy behind their HIV prevention programs.

In its original form, harm reduction, or the practice of warning drug injectors not to share needles or drug paraphernalia, dated to the 1960s. The term "harm reduction" was adopted in the 1980s and the practice expanded to giving users clean needles as well as a range of other services. The view was that a drug user need not stop entirely to reduce the damage caused by his or her drug use. Distributing clean needles to injectors has a proven track record in reducing new HIV infections in that population. Cutting unsafe sex in that population was not so successful. The reason is simple. When you give an addict a clean needle, you are helping that person do what he wants to do. There is no pleasure-increasing mechanical fix, such as a clean needle, when it comes to sex.

"You tend to find more reductions in unsafe injecting behavior than you do with unsafe sex," said Ron Stall, at the time an associate professor at the University of California at San Francisco Center for AIDS Prevention Studies, in a 1998 interview with Lesbian and Gay New York. "When you put on a condom that decreases sexual pleasure, but when you use a clean needle that increases pleasure."

While roughly 5 percent of gay and bisexual men are drug

injectors, most of the gay men who were struggling with drugs and unsafe sex were not. AIDS groups looked at the success of harm reduction among injectors and embraced it in their work with all gay men. The groups did not demand that clients abstain from drug use. They talked about engaging users "where they are at" and they did not judge them.

"It's not just around reducing intake," said Lori Elmelund, M.F.C.C. and program manager for addiction recovery services at the Los Angeles Gay and Lesbian Community Services Center, in 1998. "It's about taking care of themselves in all areas of their lives. If they choose not to eat because they are out using, we try and have planned times where they do sit down to eat . . . It's not just around reducing the destructiveness of the substance."

Programs in New York City; Seattle; Washington, D.C.; Chicago; San Francisco; and other cities adopted a harm-reduction approach. The national model was GMHC's Substance Use Counseling and Education that was founded by Elovich in 1994.

"We provide tools, we don't identify ourselves to the community, to people who are participating, as a harm reduction program or as a recovery program," Elovich said in a 1998 interview. "We describe ourselves as steps toward change and they define the change and they define what steps they take."

The problem with these programs is that they could not prove that their efforts were effective in reducing drug use or unsafe sex among their clients. By 1998, GMHC had completed a two-year evaluation of SUCE. It had enrolled over 3,100 clients in various parts of the program and the evaluation concluded with three questions. First, what degree of participation leads to changes in the client's life?; then, why some clients experience these changes and some do not?;

and, finally, "among program participants, do these 'psy-chosocial shifts' result in decreased risk for HIV infection over time?"

In 1998, reacting to that last question and the observation that GMHC currently has no data to respond to it, Elovich said, "I would actually agree. We don't. We're not a research organization. We have not done that kind of data."

Similarly, Marc Malvin, a mental health clinician at the Los Angeles Gay and Lesbian Community Services Center who ran a three-year-old men's crystal meth support group there, said in 1998, "I don't have any figures as to what the success rate is. We'd like to be able to have figures . . . It's just a question of time and dollars."

Just as these groups cannot claim success, it is not possible to say definitively that they failed. As Malvin noted, making the sort of analysis that would tie a specific prevention strategy to a specific increase or decrease in unsafe sex is expensive and time-consuming, but it appears that the best efforts of the AIDS groups had little impact on unsafe sex among these men. The "stubborn remainder" was unmoved.

We now know that sexually transmitted diseases were increasing among these gay men during the late 1990s and HIV incidence rates increased slightly in some places or remained stable at rates that were high enough to keep the epidemic growing.

In 2003, the CDC reported that HIV diagnoses in twenty-nine states grew 5.1 percent from 1999 to 2002. The agency attributed that increase to new infections among gay and bisexual men, which grew 17 percent. The data suggested that it was HIV infections among gay and bisexual men that was driving the overall increase.

"When we look by year the only risk group for which we

see an increase is men who have sex with men," Dr. Ronald O. Valdiserri, deputy director at the CDC's National Center for HIV, Sexually Transmitted Disease and Tuberculosis Prevention said in 2003. "We don't see an increase among persons who report heterosexual contact and we don't see an increase among persons who report injection drug use."

Looking at HIV "testing patterns," the CDC concluded that the increases resulted from "actual new infections and not merely a greater amount" of HIV testing.

"We do not believe that what we are seeing here is increased testing among men who have sex with men so it raises the question are we seeing more infections?" Valdiserri said. "It continues to raise serious concerns."

The twenty-nine states did not include New York, California, Illinois, Massachusetts, Washington, Texas, and the nation's capital, all of which have large gay male populations and some of which had reported outbreaks of sexually transmitted diseases among those men. In 2004, the CDC reported that syphilis and gonorrhea among gay and bisexual men appeared to be increasing though the numbers of cases never approached the totals seen in the early 1980s.

"Based on data from several cities, we believe that an increasing number of men who have sex with men are acquiring STDs," Valdiserri said. "Perhaps the most important information that we have in that regard comes from syphilis surveillance. We estimate that at least 60 percent of the primary and secondary syphilis cases reported in 2003 were among men who have sex with men."

Using data collected from the CDC's Gonococcal Isolate Surveillance Project, which tracks U.S. gonorrhea cases, syphilis case reports, and information from nine sexually transmitted disease or gay health clinics around the country, the agency said that "that an increasing number of men who have sex with men are acquiring STDs."

In 1999, 4.1 percent, on average, of the gay and bisexual men who were tested for syphilis at the "participating STD clinics" were positive for the bug compared to 10.5 percent in 2003. The recent increases in syphilis are generally attributed to more infections among gay and bisexual men.

"In the syphilis data, there is very good evidence that the increases that we have seen are due to the outbreaks of syphilis in various communities across the U.S. involving gay and bisexual men," Valdiserri said. "I think it's fair to make the general statement that after the significant declines in STDs that were observed in the late 1980s and the mid-1990s, we've started to see, particularly with syphilis, three years of increases predominantly among men who have sex with men."

The overall syphilis rate among gay and bisexual men rose "13.5 percent between 2002 and 2003, and 68 percent between 2000 and 2003," according to the CDC report. Similarly, among the "participating STD clinics," an average of 13.7 percent of the men who have sex with men tested positive for gonorrhea in 1999 compared to 15.3 percent in 2003.

HIV incidence rates among gay men in some American cities increased or remained unchanged.

In 1999, the San Francisco health department reported that the HIV incidence rate among gay men there went from 1.3 percent in 1997 to 2.6 percent in 1998 to 3.7 percent in 1999. In Seattle, public health authorities tested blood samples gathered from 1990 to 1999 and found an overall incidence of 2.4 percent among gay and bisexual men. It was highest in 1991 and 1990, at 4.9 percent, declining to 1 percent in 1994 to 1995 and increasing to 3.2 percent in 1998 and 1999. The New York City health department has reported that the incidence rate among gay men there has held at 2 to 3 percent per year from 1993 through 2003.

AIDS groups were not meeting the challenge. Asked in 2003 if the groups that have traditionally delivered HIV prevention messages to gay men were engaged in the fight against HIV, Valdiserri said, "My personal opinion is the answer to that is no. The AIDS groups are struggling with how to retool and refocus HIV prevention messages and efforts in this new era that we find ourselves in."

That view was shared by some gay community members. The HIV Forum's Kellerhouse said in 2003, "There is a philosophical piece that we have talked about. We feel that the structure that's in place, the organizations, the agencies, who have been conducting the prevention dialogue in New York City, that whatever it is they are doing isn't working. The event in some ways is a deliberate attempt to create a new dialogue and discourse about what's going on."

Similarly, in 2003, Colin Robinson, executive director of the New York State Black Gay Network, a coalition of seventeen groups in five cities across the state, said, "The passion and the individualism of HIV prevention have been lost . . . We're trying to bring meaning and agency back into HIV prevention. It's about complicating the voices that are available to us."

Robinson and Steven G. Fullwood, project director of the Black Gay and Lesbian Archive, had published a series of essays on sex, HIV, and related topics by gay and bisexual men of color have sex in *Think Again*, a book. Some of the pieces were critical of prevention efforts.

"The reality remains that many of the things that we know are effective remain in the toolbox," Robinson said. "We haven't been asking and engaging with the right questions."

Just as disturbing as the HIV incidence rates and growth in sexually transmitted diseases was the evidence, admittedly only some, that suggested that some gay men had recreated the sexual infrastructure that allowed HIV to spread in the late 1970s and early 1980s.

As syphilis was making a comeback in America, there were near simultaneous outbreaks of the bug among gay men in Western European cities and Australia. Following an outbreak of lymphogranuloma venereum, a form of chlamydia, among gay men in Belgium, France, and Sweden, health authorities in the United States reported six cases among gay men here.

In the United States, gay men in Los Angeles were confronted with an outbreak of methicillin-resistant staphylococcus aureus, or MRSA, in 2002 and 2003. By early 2004, doctors in private practice who served large numbers of gay men in New York City; Washington, D.C.; Seattle; Chicago; Denver; Boston; Houston; and Florida were reporting MRSA cases. MRSA is much easier to transmit or acquire than HIV, syphilis, or gonorrhea. Some media reports suggested that simple skin-to-skin contact could spread the bug so its rapid spread across the country is not a surprise.

As these events were happening, the AIDS groups were confronted with yet another daunting challenge. The new drugs did not just save lives, they also had an impact on the budgets of AIDS groups. Donors looked at the success of the treatments and stopped giving.

A 1999 Gallup Poll of 276 funding groups reported that the number of organizations giving a minimum of $50,000 a year to AIDS causes fell 22 percent between 1997 and 1999. The number of groups giving any money to AIDS causes fell 21 percent during that time. Forty percent of the groups that had funded AIDS groups for, at least, ten years said AIDS was no longer a priority. The poll was presented at the annual meeting of the Council on Foundations and it was reported in the *New Orleans Times-Picayune*, a newspaper.

Paul DiDonato, executive director of Funders Concerned About AIDS, told the newspaper that "long-term AIDS grantmakers may be experiencing donor fatigue" and that, as a result of the new treatments, donors "mistakenly believe that domestic progress . . . has reduced the need for philanthropic support."

Federal funding, the primary source of funding for treatment and prevention in the United States, for HIV prevention programs was slowing as well. In 1995, prevention spending, or $656 million, accounted for 10 percent of all AIDS dollars in the federal budget, according to a 2002 report from the Henry J. Kaiser Family Foundation. By 2002, that number had dropped to 7 percent, or $968 million. Federal HIV prevention spending remained flat at roughly $900 million in 2005 and 2006 and it accounted for 5 and 4 percent, respectively, of all federal AIDS funds in those years.

The population that was infected with HIV was growing, living longer, and becoming more diverse as HIV moved out of the gay community and the drug injecting population. Prevention spending was not keeping pace. At the same time, more AIDS groups sprang up to serve those diverse populations. The competition for those federal and private funds was getting tougher.

In this context of shrinking budgets, a core of gay and bisexual men whose drug use and unsafe sex represented a complex problem that AIDS groups could not solve and what had been a decade-long critique of HIV prevention efforts, the gay community was presented with a major challenge in 2005. When New York City health department announced the case of a gay man who used meth and was infected with a highly treatment-resistant strain of HIV, that caused rapid progression, the panic over meth and HIV hit a crescendo.

4

THE TRUTH ABOUT
GAY MEN

Standing before a phalanx of reporters on February 11, 2005, New York City's health commissioner announced that his department had learned of a New York City man, in his forties, who was infected with a strain of HIV that was resistant to three of the four classes of drugs used to treat the disease.

The virus could attack the man's immune system cells by attaching itself to two different receptors on those cells, a trait that is typically associated with advanced HIV infection. Most HIV can attach itself to just one receptor.

The gay man last tested negative for HIV in May of 2003, but in November 2004 he experienced flu-like symptoms and he tested positive for HIV on December 16, 2004. By January, he received an AIDS diagnosis. It usually takes years to go from HIV-positive to AIDS.

A rapid progressor infected with an aggressive, multi-drug resistant virus was troubling enough, but the man was also a meth user who reported "unprotected insertive and receptive anal intercourse with multiple partners," according to a health department alert sent to city doctors on February 11. Some press reports put the number of partners in the hundreds.

"It's a wake-up call to men who have sex with men, particularly those who may use crystal methamphetamine," Frieden said in a press statement. "Not only are we seeing syphilis and a rare sexually transmitted disease, lymphogranuloma venereum, among these men, now we've identified this strain of HIV that is difficult or impossible to treat and which appears to progress rapidly to AIDS."

The health department learned of the case from the Aaron Diamond AIDS Research Center in late January and, at first, department staff questioned whether the case was significant.

"Our decision process in this was, 'Is this real? Is this a real phenomena?'" Frieden said at a March 3 town meeting organized by the HIV Forum. "We were skeptical about it."

Frieden said that when the department was confident that the case might be "a harbinger of increasing drug resistance," it held the February 11 press conference to announce the case and that may have prevented other infections.

"I think our going public with it made it less likely that [the virus] will be widely disseminated," Frieden told the audience of roughly 350 that had gathered at an auditorium on a local college campus. "We did not make this announcement to increase fear. We made this announcement because we felt we had a responsibility."

The news certainly did inspire fear in some gay men. Following Frieden's announcement, the *New York Times* quoted Edsel Gonzalez, a thirty-year-old business owner from South Beach, saying he was "absolutely worried about this . . . It seems like we're moving backwards in the fight against AIDS."

The press coverage was extensive and predictably fevered.

The case earned international news coverage with the virus variously described as an "AIDS Super Bug," a "frightening, never-before-seen superstrain," and a "new strain of the AIDS virus that swiftly causes disease and resists virtually all anti-HIV drugs." GMHC's *Treatment News*, a bi-monthly journal, noted one headline in an international newspaper that read "New AIDS Peril Puts America on High Alert."

Just as earlier press coverage had launched and driven debates about HIV prevention in the gay community, the news of a supposedly new strain resulted in harsh condemnations, calls for new actions against HIV, and, now, statements that expressed hopelessness that the epidemic would ever end.

Charles Kaiser, author of *The Gay Metropolis*, told the *New York Times* that "Gay men do not have the right to spread a debilitating and often fatal disease . . . A person who is HIV positive has no more right to unprotected intercourse than he has the right to put a bullet through another person's head." Kaiser made similar comments in the *Washington Post*.

The same *Times* article that cited Kaiser, titled "Gays Debate Radical Steps to Curb Unsafe Sex," suggested that some in the gay community were considering more aggressive steps to prevent the spread of HIV though it did not quote anyone who actually proposed these steps.

"They want to track down those who knowingly engage in risky behavior and try to stop them before they can infect others," the article read. "Although gay advocates and health care workers are just beginning to talk about how this might be done, it could involve showing up at places where impromptu sex parties happen and confronting the participants. Or it might mean infiltrating Web sites that promote gay hookups and thwarting liaisons involving crystal meth . . . Other ideas include collaborating with health officials in tracking down the partners of those newly infected with HIV."

Writing in his weekly column, Savage suggested that anyone who infects another person with HIV be required to pay for the treatment of that second person.

"Infect someone with HIV out of malice or negligence and the state will come after you for half the cost of the meds the person you infected is going to need," Savage wrote. "Once a few dozen men in New York City, San Francisco, Toronto, Los Angeles, Chicago, Miami, and Vancouver are having their wages docked for drug-support payments, other gay men will be a lot more careful about not spreading HIV. Trojan won't be able to make condoms fast enough."

In an April issue of *New York* magazine Savage said, "There's a great deal of anger and frustration among gays and lesbians at the never-ending, nonstop coddling and compassion campaign that passes for HIV prevention . . . There will be no sympathy when this happens to us again. We are not going to be the baby harp seals the way we were in the 1980s and 1990s. We picked up the same gun and said, 'I hope it's not loaded this time,' and pulled the trigger again. And I'm gay, imagine how straight people feel."

The atmosphere was such that GMHC, which for years had been consistently careful and moderate in its comments on HIV prevention, opposed Savage's proposal, not because it was wrong, but because it was unworkable.

"We find ourselves at a time where the idea of holding people accountable, of building consequences into behavior choices, may be needed to help change the paradigm," Oliveira told Savage. "We certainly appreciate the element of justice in your idea. It could act as a deterrent, and that would be helpful. The difficulty is that it would be impractical to implement. It would require some kind of a determination process and the pitfall would be a lot of he said/he said situations."

Most striking was the defeatism, perhaps even nihilism, that emerged following the announcement. Rotello told the *Times* that gay men would not change until they experienced the death and terror that characterized the AIDS epidemic in the early 1980s.

"People are not going to modify their sexual habits in ways that are difficult or unpleasant until they see their friends dying again," he said. "And to me that's just an unbelievably depressing thought."

Kramer, who had given a gloomy, misery-filled speech in November in New York City, titled "The Tragedy of Today's Gays" in which he said that gay men were "murdering each other" when they had sex without condoms in the early years of the AIDS epidemic and that they continued that behavior today, responded to the news reports on the "AIDS Super Bug" by declaring that that HIV prevention had never worked.

"Even in the days of the worst infections, no amount of prevention seemed to work, and that's probably the scariest thing of all," Kramer told the *Times*.

The press brought little skepticism to bear on the science behind the case despite the number of researchers who were publicly expressing doubts. Among the doubters was Dr. Robert C. Gallo, director of the Institute of Human Virology and Division of Basic Science at the University of Maryland Biotechnology Institute and a co-discoverer of HIV.

"The word would be greater than skepticism," Gallo told *Gay City News*. "There is zero evidence at this time that this is super-HIV. We've had claims of super-HIV in the past. None have been borne out."

Dr. John P. Moore, a professor of microbiology and immunology at the Weill Medical College of Cornell University, shared Gallo's view.

"Firstly, it's not new that multi-drug resistant viruses are around," Moore said. "It's also not new that rapidly progressing viruses are around. It's also not new that you can have the two traits in one individual."

As to the concern that the New York City man may have passed the bug to his sex partners, Gallo and Moore said that the mutations that create drug resistance in HIV often result in a virus that is less effective at infecting others. The bug may be "a super wimpy virus from the transmission perspective," Moore said.

"Transmission of multi-drug resistant viruses is relatively inefficient," Moore said. "I would take this more seriously if there was a cluster because it would prove that the virus is transmissible."

As months passed, the case grew less compelling as new articles, mostly in the gay press and medical journals, disclosed new facts. With each disclosure, the New York City health department grew more tightlipped.

At the March 3 town meeting, the crowd learned that the man was responding to treatment. Dr. Lawrence G. Hitzeman, an attending physician at Cabrini Medical Center who spoke with the man's doctor, said that the man's viral load, a measure of the amount of virus in his blood, went from over 600,000 to 4,000 after being treated with four drugs. Hitzeman said that the drop was "significant," but it could take three to six months to determine if his response to treatment was "durable." The man's T-cell count, a measure of his immune system health, was still very low at forty-eight. A normal T-cell count ranges from 700 to 1,200. *New York* magazine reported in April that the man had returned to work.

Then in the June 4 issue of *The Lancet*, a British medical journal, Geoffrey S. Gottlieb and David C. Nickle, two University of Washington researchers, raised the possibility that a dual infection was responsible for the New York City case.

An infection with more than one strain of HIV would explain the man's rapid progression from HIV-positive to AIDS because dual infections are associated with that type of progression. A dual infection would also explain why no second case had been found. The likelihood that the New York City man, or any dually infected person, could infect a second person with all of the HIV strains he or she is infected with is very low.

In his response in The Lancet to Gottlieb and Nickle, Dr. Martin Markowitz, the clinical director at the Aaron Diamond center who reported the case to the health department, wrote, "We wholeheartedly agree with Geoffrey Gottlieb and David Nickle. Indeed we cannot rule out the possibility of dual infection or superinfection in this case, but we are exploring these possibilities."

After each revelation, the city health department would only say, "The investigation remains ongoing" and by July 27 a department press statement read, "The source of infection for the patient announced in February cannot be determined with available information."

The agency had ordered thirty-nine testing labs across the country to report any cases found between June 1, 2004, and June 30, 2005, that matched or were similar to the February case. On July 27, the agency reported only that it had unearthed three people "with strains of HIV that are equally closely related to the strain of the case announced in February." A national search for a second case had produced no match.

In retrospect, this case looked less like a meth-fueled outbreak of virulent, drug-resistant HIV and, perhaps, more like a sad story of one gay man who had the misfortune to get infected with more than one strain of HIV, at least one of which was highly drug-resistant.

The press, generally, paid far less attention to the later developments that tended to undercut the "AIDS Super Bug" theme. With most of their information coming from the earlier stories, it is understandable that some, perhaps many, gay men came to believe that a new strain of virulent, drug-resistant HIV threatened their health and their lives.

In as much as the announcement inspired fear, it also made some in the gay and AIDS communities very angry. Some questioned the science and the assertion that this case represented a new strain or even a new phenomenon.

The Community HIV/AIDS Mobilization Project, a New York City AIDS group, issued a press release responding to Frieden's announcement that pointed out that "two cases of rapidly-progressing virus resistant to three classes of HIV drugs" had been reported in Vancouver in 2001.

"What became of that was not a widespread multi-drug resistant virus epidemic," said Julie Davids, CHAMP's executive director. "Unless there is something they aren't telling us, this isn't new. It isn't accurate to say this hasn't happened before; it has."

Just as earlier debates concerning gay men and HIV were perceived by some as little more than attacks on gay male sexuality, Davids said that the announcement could stigmatize gay men.

"I think one of the harms is pointing fingers at gay men instead of pointing resources," she said. "In the history of the AIDS crisis, we've always had a scapegoat."

In a press statement sent to *Gay City News*, Martin Delaney, the founding director of Project Inform, a San Francisco AIDS group, wrote, "I have no disagreement about the need for the gay community to address the issues of crystal meth abuse and related failures to protect our community and each other from HIV. I do not believe, however, that this conversation should be driven by what is only a scientific anecdote. Many of the statements made about the New York patient were and remain uncertain and unproven."

Lost in the media hype over an "AIDS Super Bug" was the real problem—that portion of the gay male community that had abandoned or never practiced safe sex. Also lost was that population of gay men who had not given up safe sex or had altered their behavior to reduce their risk of infection. The most dramatic, recent example of this second group came out of San Francisco and Los Angeles.

A 2005 CDC study of 1,767 gay and bisexual men in five American cities, including the two West Coast cities, reported an annual rate of new HIV infections of 1.2 percent among the San Francisco men and 1.4 percent among the Los Angeles men. The good news caught public health officials in San Francisco by surprise where the most recent estimate of HIV incidence among gay men there was 2.2 percent. In a news report, they were described as "scrambling" to explain the decline.

A number of reasons were offered for the decline in media reports, but none suggested that part of the reason may be that gay men are having safe sex. Gay men who are sexually active and safe are often ignored in discussions about sex and

HIV in favor of newer or more provocative topics. A *New York Times* story on the decrease in HIV incidence among gay men in San Francisco suggested it was due entirely to sero-sorting, or the practice of selecting sex partners according to their HIV status. Doubtless there are multiple reasons for the declines in San Francisco and Los Angeles and among them is that plenty of gay men have safe sex.

In 2004, Jeffrey T. Parsons, a psychology professor at Hunter College and the director of CHEST, made the point that not every gay man who has sex with many partners is meth-addicted and sexually compulsive.

"There are perfectly, psychologically healthy men out there who are having a lot of sex and are safe and enjoying it," Parsons said.

Looking at the declines in sexually transmitted diseases among gay men dating back to the early 1980s, MHRA's Chiasson made a similar observation.

"Although we've seen a big increase in syphilis recently it's nowhere near where it was twenty years ago," she said in 2004. "It does suggest that there have been big changes in behavior. More people may be using condoms, more people may be having fewer partners, more people may be having sequential versus concurrent partners."

The phrase "sequential versus concurrent partners" refers to the practice of having multiple sex partners, but one at a time each for a period of time as opposed to having sex with many different men at roughly the same time. Having sequential partners can contribute to reducing the spread of HIV. To illustrate this, Rotello used two hypothetical men in *Sexual Ecology*.

Both men have twelve partners a year and the same amount and type of sex with those men. One man has one partner a month, in sequence, going from partner one through twelve. The second man travels between all twelve sex partners throughout the year. If both men become infected in October, the man with sequential partners can potentially infect two men while the man with concurrent partners can infect twelve men. The difference is significant.

Gay men are also taking other steps to reduce the risk of acquiring HIV and certainly sero-sorting is one of them. With sero-sorting, HIV-negative men select HIV-negative sex partners and achieve a zero risk of HIV infection. Similarly, HIV-positive men select HIV-positive partners. There is an ongoing debate in the gay community about the risk of re-infection when two positive men have unprotected sex.

Sero-sorting can also mean altering one's sexual behavior depending on the HIV status of one's sex partner. A recent CHEST study showed clear evidence of sero-sorting among its 174 sexually active participants. Overall, men in the study who were uninfected had much less sex, either anal or oral, with casual partners they knew to be positive.

Less than 1 percent of the 138 HIV-negative men in that study reported having receptive oral sex to ejaculation when they were having sex with an HIV-positive partner and 1.4 percent of the negative men reported receptive anal sex to ejaculation when their partner was positive.

Those same negative men reported different behavior when their partner was uninfected. Just under 24 percent of the negative men reported receptive oral sex to ejaculation with a negative partner and just under 11 percent reported receptive anal sex to ejaculation with a negative partner. Across the board, the study clearly showed that the negative men altered their behavior when they knew their partner was infected.

The thirty-six positive men also changed their behavior depending on their partner's HIV status. Just over 22 percent reported being the top during oral sex to ejaculation when their partner was also positive, but only 11 percent reported that behavior when their partner was negative. Eighteen percent topped during anal sex with ejaculation with a positive partner, but only 4.5 percent of the positive men reported that behavior with a negative partner. Other studies have shown similar results.

A small 2003 study of forty-three HIV-positive men in San Francisco reported sero-sorting in that population. These men had sex with both negative and positive partners, but during bareback sex the negative men were the receptive partners just 7 percent of the time. When they knew their partner was also positive, they practiced bareback sex 91 percent of the time.

In a 1997 analysis published in *AIDS and Behavior*, a journal, Dr. Sally M. Blower, a professor of biomathematics at the University of California at Los Angeles, discussed the results of a 1995 study in which she showed that sex between young gay men in San Francisco and older gay men, a population with higher HIV prevalence, had led to more infections among the younger gay men.

In that study, whether a participant chose a negative or positive partner was as important as whether the study participant had anal sex, the riskiest type of sex. Sexual partner selection "has been as important a risk factor for HIV as having multiple receptive anal intercourse partners," Blower wrote.

Sero-sorting is an imperfect method in that it relies on a sex partner knowing his status and being honest about it.

"You can have a situation where somebody thinks they are engaged in sero-sorting, but because the other person doesn't

know their status or isn't honest then you have the opportunity for transmission," Parsons said.

Sero-sorting also assumes that men discuss their status with
their partners. They do not always do that. The 2003 San
Francisco study reported that in the 176 "unique partner-
ships," or sexual encounters, "sero-disclosure was only
reported" in half.

A 2003 study of syphilis among gay men in New York City
showed even less conversation. That study looked at the
sexual behavior, drug use, and HIV rates among 264 men.
Among its conclusions was that the men were not discussing
HIV at all let alone disclosing their status.

"People aren't talking about [HIV]," said Dr. Susan Blank,
assistant commissioner of the New York City health department's Bureau of Sexually Transmitted Disease Control and
the study's author. "They are just having sex with other people
without talking about it."

All of the men in the syphilis study were engaging in high-
risk behavior.

"What we found was that many [men who have sex with
men] were engaging in high-risk sexual behaviors," Blank
said. "Specifically that meant sex with multiple, anonymous
partners, unprotected anal intercourse, barebacking, recre-
ational drug use before sex and not discussing HIV status
prior to sex with a partner."

A Seattle study found only some discussion of HIV
among gay and bisexual men. The health department there
interviewed 34 HIV-positive gay men and 115 HIV-
negative gay men in 2003 and found that while they were
having some discussions about HIV status with their sex
partners those conversations were often incomplete. While
59 percent talked about HIV with their partners, only 39

percent actually knew their partner's HIV status before having anal sex.

Even with its flaws, sero-sorting can still reduce the risk of HIV infection. There have been other profound changes in the gay community that have made it much harder for HIV to thrive there and one is the widespread use of anti-HIV drugs.

Those drugs can reduce the amount of virus in a person's body to an undetectable level and, more than any other factor, the amount of virus, or viral load, determines how infectious a person is. As more HIV-positive gay men take these drugs, the amount of virus in the community, or "community viral load" as one researcher put it, is reduced. There is simply less virus available to infect people.

"There is no question that it lowers viral load," said Chiasson. "[Viral load] is the strongest correlation with transmission. You would assume that it has got to be having some impact."

In 2004, the CDC's Valdiserri said, "The effectiveness of treatments is extremely important. If enough people are treated and the frequency of sexual behavior is stable, there will be a decrease."

In a 2003 study published in *AIDS Reviews*, a journal, Blower wrote that with sustained reductions in unsafe sex and continued use of anti-HIV drugs could end the epidemic though that would take many years.

"Modeling predictions have been made for the San Francisco gay community of the potential epidemic-level effects of [anti-retroviral therapy] (ART) in terms of HIV infections prevented and AIDS deaths averted," Blower wrote. "These analyses have shown that a high usage of ART (treating 50 percent to 90 percent of HIV-infected persons) substantially decreases the annual AIDS death rate, by increasing survival, and also substantially reduces the transmission rate, by reducing average viral load . . . Furthermore, it has been shown that a high usage of ART, treating 50 percent to 90 percent of HIV-infected individuals, coupled with reductions in risky behavior could result in the eradication of HIV epi-demics, even those of high prevalence. However, epidemic eradication would take many decades."

The anti-HIV drugs are a powerful influence on the course of the epidemic and then there have been some fundamental cultural shifts in the gay community that may have con-tributed to a reduction in the spread of HIV among gay men. The most obvious one is marriage and its implied monogamy.

In the late 1970s and early 1980s, the dominant ethos was sexual liberation. Same-sex marriage was rarely pursued or even discussed. While there are still community members who hold a liberationist view—it is probably more accurate to say that they oppose the assimilation into the wider culture that marriage would bring—but their point of view has been marginalized. Perhaps due to recent court victories, marriage now dominates queer discourse.

In a 2003 Harris Interactive Poll of 748 lesbian, gay, bisexual, and transgender adults, 78 percent responded affir-matively when asked, "If you were in a committed relation-ship, would you personally want to obtain a civil marriage license?" Similarly, in an exit poll taken during the 2004 gen-eral election, 51 percent of gay or lesbian voters said that they should be allowed to marry. Thirty-one percent said that they should be allowed to have civil unions, but not marriages. The pursuit of marriage certainly suggests that some gay male cou-ples are in monogamous relationships.

The support for the pursuit of marriage may grow stronger over time. In a 2005 analysis of the Harris and exit poll data,

Kenneth Sherrill, a professor of political science at Hunter College, and Patrick J. Egan, a Ph.D. candidate in political science at the University of California at Berkeley, noted that the support for same-sex marriage among gay men and lesbians split along generational lines with younger community members being more likely to back it. As that younger generation moves into leadership positions, it is likely that marriage will become more important in the community.

"In sum, these results suggest that a strong generational effect may be in place among LGBTs that will lead same-sex marriage to become an issue of steadily increasing priority," the authors wrote in *Political Science & Politics*, a journal that is published by the American Political Science Association. Marriage is not the only indicator of changed community norms.

There are, at least, five twelve-step programs operating in the United States today that assist their members in overcoming what they identify as sexually compulsive behavior. All of those groups list meetings that are held at gay and lesbian community organizations. In some cities, such as New York, a substantial number of their meetings are held at gay-identified institutions. For a segment of the lesbian and gay community, the unbridled sexuality that was once seen as a hallmark of a liberation movement has become a problem that requires the assistance of a program and a higher power.

Taken together, the pursuit of same-sex marriage and the rise of these twelve-step groups show clear shift among some gay and lesbian community members. This is not to say that the sexuality of sexual liberation has been abandoned. On the contrary, it is alive and well, but it is tempered by other community values.

"Relationships are more common now," Parsons said. "They are more accepted . . . I think what's happened in the community is that we have different norms. We have some norms that are very opposed to risky sex and having lots of partners. There are other norms that support barebacking and lots of partners."

All of these influences, safe sex, the data on sero-sorting, the effect of treatment, and the changes in gay male culture should also inform the community's response to crystal meth. Obviously, some practices are working to keep some gay men safe. One response might be to assess what those are and, if possible, determine if and how they could be taught to or used by the men who are not being safe. Instead, what was seen in the "AIDS Super Bug" coverage was hysteria.

Responding to the "AIDS Super Bug" revelations, community leaders and commentators, some of them are quite intelligent and informed, simply obliterated those portions of gay community history that showed that some gay men had taken steps to end or reduce their risk of becoming infected. Others called for punitive measures or establishing what appeared to be community vigilantes to patrol sex clubs and parties.

The gay community has seen this hysteria before. It was present when otherwise thoughtful leaders announced in 1994 that "prevention had failed" or that there was a "crisis of new infections" among gay men. It was present in the blame focused on barebackers and men on the "down low" or the attention given to "bug chasers" and "gift givers." The latter two phenomena are little more than urban legends.

All of these responses have shown a kind of blindness as activists and commentators have focused on a single element of the epidemic rather survey the entire landscape.

We saw this in 1996 when Sullivan looked at just one part of the gay male community and declared that the plague was ended. The leaders in the gay men's health movement, such as

Rofes, made a similar mistake. As the name of their movement suggests, they were clearly well intended and gay men were at the heart of their agenda. They correctly noted that the sense of crisis that had characterized AIDS in the 1980s had passed and they understood the effect of the anti-HIV drugs. They failed to take any substantive note of their peers who were not staying safe.

Some of those who opposed Sullivan and Rofes, such as Signorile and Rotello, might also have overstated the threat that viral resistance to those anti-HIV drugs posed to gay men.

What the data tells us is that what Lingua Franca called the "stubborn remainder" has been with us since the first days of the AIDS epidemic and the behavior of those men appears to have been largely unaffected by the debating, the press reports, and the hand-wringing that has occurred in the gay community since those first days.

That same hysteria that was exhibited in response to earlier "crises" is certainly a part of the response to crystal use among gay men. It is apparent in some of the town meetings, the anti-crystal posters, and news reports, in the gay and mainstream press, on meth and gay men. The same blindness is apparent as well.

At a June 2004 conference on meth held in New York City, Sabina Hirshfield, an MHRA researcher, presented data from a national survey of gay and bisexual men, some of whom were meth users. In the 2002 survey of 2,916 men, 6 percent reported using meth and 82 percent of them, or about 145 men, reported having unprotected anal sex at least once in the prior six months. Among the men who did not report crystal use, 55 percent, or roughly fifteen hundred men, reported having had unprotected anal sex.

All of these men, those who used meth and those who did

not, were having lots of sex. Asked how many partners they had in the six months before taking the survey, 93 percent of the crystal users had two to over one hundred partners, but 79 percent of the men who did not use crystal also fell into that range.

The combination of unsafe sex and lots of partners is clearly bad news, but when Hirshfield was asked by one audience member if her data showed a group of non-crystal users who were not staying safe, other audience members hit the roof. These were staffers from leading AIDS groups and public health agencies. As they looked at the numbers that told them that some gay men who did not use meth were struggling with safe sex, they insisted that these men only had a "slip up" or that they had had unsafe sex with a primary partner whose HIV status they knew. It was only the men who used meth who were the problem. In a 2004 interview with *Out*, Hirshfield disagreed.

"I think it is really a lot of people who are having high-risk sex," she said.

The simple truth is that the AIDS epidemic among gay men, like all epidemics in any population, has always been a complex interaction of the virus with various behaviors, including sex and drug-taking behaviors, and, more recently, with anti-HIV drugs. The gay community, more often than not, has opted to reduce this interaction to a single cause.

"I think what we want as a community is to find a single X factor to explain what is going on," Halkitis told *Out* in 2004. "We lose the big picture, we lose the landscape because we are focused on one of the trees."

The single X factor, crystal in this case, certainly is contributing to the spread of HIV among gay men.

A 2005 study in San Francisco tested 2,991 gay men who visited that city's sexually transmitted disease clinic in 2000 and 2001. Among the 290 men who reported meth use the HIV incidence rate was 6.3 percent annually. That rate was 2.1 percent annually among the remaining 2,701 who said they did not use the drug.

The virus had to overcome some significant obstacles to get to that rate. Large numbers of HIV-positive, gay men in San Francisco are taking anti-HIV drugs, and safe sex and sero-sorting are common there, and, as America saw in 2004, when that city's mayor ordered San Francisco's marriage bureau to issue licenses to same-sex couples, thousands of gay and lesbian couples got married there. Despite these influences, the HIV incidence rate among those meth users hit a number that has not been seen in San Francisco since the early 1980s.

Meth, however, is not the only factor and that is a source of frustration for some researchers. At the 2004 meth conference, Hunter College's Parsons was shaking his head following a presentation he gave. His community had become obsessed with another X factor. Parsons told *Out* that crystal is dangerous and it "should have a lot of the focus, but it shouldn't have the exclusive focus." Other drugs are dangerous as well.

"We're still seeing a relationship between the use of other drugs and unsafe sex and a relationship between the use of alcohol and unsafe sex," he told the magazine.

While the 2002 Hunter College study of 786 gay and bisexual men found crystal users were 3.5 times more likely to report unprotected anal sex with a partner of a different HIV status in the ninety days before taking the survey than men who did not use crystal it also found that men who used other "club drugs" were also being unsafe.

Those who used GHB were just over three times more likely to report unprotected anal sex. Cocaine, ecstasy, or Special K users were roughly 2.5 times more likely to report that unsafe behavior than men who did not use those drugs. Men who used alcohol were 1.5 times more likely to report that behavior than non-drinkers. When one considers that 46 percent of the sample, or 314 men, reported combining alcohol and sex compared to the 6 percent of the sample, or 47 men, who combined crystal and sex, certainly a reasonable person would be as concerned about the men who drank. Overall, whether they were HIV-positive or negative, men who had unprotected anal sex with a partner of a different HIV status were more likely to use club drugs, the survey concluded.

"Unsafe sex is going on among those who are using crystal and among those who don't use crystal," Parsons said.

A 2005 study published in *AIDS*, a journal, looked at the sex lives and drug use of 1,168 gay and bisexual men in New York City and San Francisco from 1999 to 2001 and found that men who used any type of speed were three times more likely than non-users to engage in unprotected receptive anal sex with an HIV-positive casual partner and those who used meth were 5.3 times more likely to engage in that behavior.

This was also true with other drugs. Men who used Special K were nearly four times more likely than non-users to engage unprotected receptive anal sex with an HIV-positive casual partner and GHB users were 4.6 times more likely to engage in that behavior.

The EXPLORE study, which was published in the *American Journal of Public Health* in 2003, concluded, "Men who reported having used marijuana, poppers, hallucinogens, cocaine, or amphetamines in the six months before study enrollment were significantly more likely than men who did not use such drugs to report unprotected anal sex during that same period, regardless of the HIV sero-status of their partners."

The study authors noted that drinking and unsafe sex was particularly important especially "heavy alcohol use" which they defined as four drinks per day or "an amount equal to six drinks per occasion." Just over 26 percent of the sample drank at least three days a week in the six months before the study and 10.6 percent were heavy drinkers.

"Heavy alcohol use was significantly associated with unprotected receptive anal sex with partners of unknown status and partners positive for HIV antibodies, as well as with unprotected insertive anal sex with partners of unknown status," they wrote.

A number of studies have implicated drug and alcohol use among gay and bisexual men in unsafe sex.

"We're seeing a problem not just because of crystal, but because of the drug problem overall," Halkitis told Out. "It's the bigger drug picture that is the problem here."

The exclusive focus on crystal also misunderstands the nature of crystal use among gay men. Those men are typically poly-drug users.

The NYU center study that assessed the club drug use and sex lives of 450 men found that among the men who reported using meth in their first interview for the study, only 7.9 percent used crystal exclusively. All the other meth users combined meth with anywhere from one to more than four other drugs.

Another study, published in 2005 and done by researchers at the University of California at San Diego, surveyed 261 HIV-positive, gay, and bisexual men who used crystal. Just 5 percent reported using only meth in the two months prior to the study. Thirty-one percent of the men were "light poly-drug users" who used meth, marijuana, and poppers and 64 percent were "heavy poly-drug users" who used meth, cocaine, heroin, hallucinogens, and Special K.

It is true that men who use crystal tend to have more sex partners and more unsafe sex than men who do not use the drug, but if these poly-drug users stopped using crystal today that does not mean they would stop having unsafe sex nor does it mean that they would stop using other drugs. On the contrary, it is likely that they would still use and they would continue to have unsafe sex. This is likely due to the motivations that underlie their drug use.

In the seroconvert study done by Halkitis, those men were using the drug to ease feelings of loneliness or depression. The seroconverts were more likely to report using meth to avoid "unpleasant emotions," "physical discomfort," or conflict with others than the HIV-negative meth users. The seroconverts also said they used meth to have "pleasant times with others" more than the negative men.

"The implication is that these may be men who are so dependent on this drug to be with other men that when they are with those men they lose all inhibitions," Halkitis said. "That feeling of isolation and depression are absolutely key."

In his 1997 study, Gorman quoted one gay man who spoke to this point. He had not used meth in four years, but had recently decided to start using again.

"I don't want to tell you that for four years I didn't do any crystal at all, but for four years I didn't have any sex at all," he said. "So part of the loneliness comes in . . . everything just kind of stopped . . . and I thought, you know what? I didn't stop doing everything to be unhappy or to be lonely. So right or wrong, I don't care what anybody thinks, I'm going to make this decision [to use again] because I want to. This is how I want the end of my life to look like."

The social aspects of the drug use cannot and should not be discounted. Some former meth users will describe the days-long binges that they engaged in that involved not only using the drug, having sex, but also times when they were sitting in the private home or club where the party was taking place and engaging in conversation with other men. For some, that interaction was as valuable as the drug use and the sex.

For others, the sex itself is the point of taking that drug. Another Gorman informant made this point in an interview.

"And then it became like a sex thing," he said. "Because I discovered quite by accident that crystal plus sex equals, oh my God. I mean, you know, you thought it was good before when you were sober . . . It's like I didn't even think that a human body would have the capacity to create those sort of sensations."

Then the disinhibiting effect of crystal described by Halkitis may have everything to do with why the men use the drugs. The high itself is pleasant and then, because they are high, they can engage in unprotected sex without their sober mind making them feel threatened or worried about any possible consequences that could result from that sex.

In 1999, Ostrow theorized that the goal of drug use, not just crystal use, among some gay men was to have unprotected sex and he developed a program, called the Awareness Intervention for Men, that was intended to make them aware of the "scenario" they were playing out.

"The goal of the AIM intervention is get the men to recognize this," Ostrow said in 1999. "Goal number two is to get them to recognize what it is they are really after and, number three, is to help them develop a new set of scenarios."

Some gay men who use meth may be contending with serious mental illness, such as major depression or bipolar disorder, and their drug use may be a form of self-medication.

A 2004 study from the University of California at San Diego

surveyed 194 HIV-positive gay and bisexual men who used meth. Sixty percent had been under a psychiatrist's care at some time, 31 percent were taking psychiatric medications at the time of the study, and 52 percent had received a psychiatric diagnosis. Among those who had received a diagnosis, depression was the most common diagnosis at 66 percent, followed by bipolar disorder at 21 percent, followed by anxiety at 5 percent.

Some researchers have argued against the notion that drug and alcohol use among people with serious mental illness is a form of self-medication. Instead, they have advanced a theory that the drug use makes it possible for a mentally ill person to join a social setting, such as a bar or party, where he or she can interact with others and overcome the isolation that is often part of mental illness. In the context of gay men and meth this would make sense. Crystal becomes the ticket that gets a man into an environment where he can have sex with and engage socially with his peers.

For yet another group of men, the so-called barebackers, the drugs and the unsafe sex are part of a culture that rejects safe sex as dull and embraces sexual adventurism.

A 2002 NYU center study of 518 gay and bisexual men in New York City found that 448 knew the term barebacking and 45.5 percent, or 204, of these men reported having had bareback sex in the three months prior to participating in the study. Of the 448 men, 70 percent said that gay men are more likely to be using "club drugs," such as crystal meth, GHB, or ecstasy, if they are having bareback sex. Many of the men offered multiple reasons for the emergence of barebacking. Forty-nine percent said the practice had emerged because of "boring" safe-sex campaigns; 48 percent said the anti-HIV drugs had contributed; 46 percent said AIDS fatigue was a cause; and 40 percent described barebacking as a "sexual and cultural phenomenon."

Generally, the men reported that barebacking was beneficial because it increased feelings of intimacy and romance. Bareback sex also affirmed their sense of masculinity.

Altogether, and perhaps even individually, the crystal high, the sex, and the social aspects of crystal use serve as powerful motivators and rewards for meth users. While the poster campaigns that have gone up around the nation may keep some men from starting to use crystal and they may move occasional users to stop, it is hard to imagine that they will ever change the minds of the serious users. It is equally hard to conceive of the heated rhetoric concerning meth that has appeared in some press reports will make a difference in the lives of committed crystal users. Like many other drugs, both legal and illegal, meth's allure is so strong in so many ways.

The discourse on crystal and gay men has also failed to note that even within the population of crystal users there are different types or groups of users who are living very different lives.

There are those in the gay community and in public health agencies who would disagree, but the best data we have suggests that there are gay men who use crystal occasionally and, presumably, they enjoy it.

The 2004 study of one thousand gay men by the Massachusetts health department found that 10 percent reported using meth at least once in the prior year while 2 percent said they used the drug once a week. The 2001 Chicago study put meth use among gay men there at 7 percent with just 2 percent reporting monthly use. Most of the men in these two studies are not regular users. These data suggest that most of these men used the drug once or only now and again.

In the 1999 NYU center study of forty-nine gay and bisexual New York City men who used crystal, 67 percent used crystal less than once a week during the three months prior to participating in the study. Just over 18 percent reported using meth once or twice a week and 14 percent used the drug more than twice a week.

It must be said that there are dangers even in occasional meth use. The drug itself can be very damaging to the body and to the brain in particular. Then, if an occasional user is having sex in that population of men who use frequently, because HIV prevalence tends to be higher among those men, the chances of encountering an HIV-positive sex partner are increased. The recent HIV incidence data out of San Francisco also suggests that when having sex in the crystal using population, the chances of encountering a sex partner who is newly infected, and highly infectious, are also increased. Still, it may be possible that a gay man who thoughtfully plans his meth use and sex, and adheres to that plan, can avoid these problems.

Then there are demographic or sociological differences even among those men who are frequent or regular meth users.

The 2004 study from the University of California at San Diego compared meth injectors to non-injectors. The injectors reported different motivations for using the drug. They were "significantly more likely than non-injectors to report" using meth "to cope with mood," "to cope with HIV symptoms," and "to feel more self-confident," though the number of non-injectors who reported these motivations was not small.

The injectors had been using the drug for more years, they used it for more days when they got high, and they used more of the drug during binges. They also reported more financial problems, family issues, violence, and legal problems. The injectors were convicted of felonies twice as often as the non-injectors.

The 1997 Gorman study identified at least seven subgroups that were using meth in Seattle. These included gay men who attended circuit parties, "men whose sexual/drug focus appears to center on activities in gay baths and sex clubs," a transgender group, a group involved with "several young adult/youth clubs and street scenes," "a population of AIDS-infected men" who use meth and other drugs "to self-medicate the effects of HIV," middle-class gay men who are "weekend users," and gay men who live in the Seattle suburbs and party with crystal in the city. Gorman noted that the men with AIDS "appear to be quite indigent, transient, and/or homeless; they also report co-existing mental health problems such as depression."

What this data means is that the gay community has to respond with multiple strategies and interventions. All of these groups are different, they use meth in different ways and settings, for different reasons, and what would be an appropriate response to one group might be useless to another.

The "weekend users" might find instruction on how the plan their weekend use valuable. They need to decide in advance how much meth they will use, what activities, sexual or otherwise, they will or will not participate in, when they will eat, when they will take medications, if they are on medication, and so on. The users who attend circuit parties, gay baths, and sex clubs could use similar help.

Clearly, a population of people with AIDS who use meth are homeless, and contending with "co-existing mental health problems" need far more than information on how to mitigate the harm that meth can cause. They need housing, food, and medical care to name just a few things.

In a perfect world, we would see gay community organizations using with a variety of interventions and strategies. Not only are government and private funds limited, some of the strategies that these groups might use have long been contested.

Those safe-sex and drug interventions that target gay men have also been under assault, to varying degrees, since they first appeared.

In 1987, Helms, now the former U.S. Senator, objected to a sexually explicit safe-sex pamphlet produced by GMHC using private funds. The agency was also receiving federal funds at the time. A Helms-sponsored bill banned using federal money for materials that "promote or encourage, directly or indirectly, homosexual sexual activities." It easily passed the House and Senate. GMHC sued and those restrictions were struck down in 1992.

Instead, the federal government put in place new rules for CDC-funded HIV prevention programs that required that such materials include "information about the harmful effects of promiscuous sexual activity and intravenous substance abuse, and the benefits of abstaining from such activities" and that no funds be used to "promote or encourage, directly, homosexual or heterosexual sexual activity or intravenous substance abuse." The materials also cannot be obscene as that is defined under federal law.

Obscenity weighs whether "the average person, applying contemporary community standards," would see the material as appealing to the "prurient interest," depicting sex in a "patently offensive way," and lacking in "serious literary, artistic, political, or scientific value."

The political pressures on AIDS groups eased during the Clinton administration, but with the Republican Party holding the executive and legislative branches of the federal government, those attacks have begun again.

In 2001, the Bush administration launched a series of audits into spending at AIDS groups across the country. These audits often came at the request of right-wing members of Congress who are allied with conservative groups that have called for cuts in federal AIDS spending.

In 2004, the Bush administration proposed new guidelines that would require AIDS groups to pre-clear all their CDC-funded HIV prevention materials with a review panel to be created by their state or local health department. Previously, AIDS groups created their own review panels that included a representative from their state or local health department.

While AIDS groups in such places as New York City and San Francisco were confident their materials would pass such panels, the concern was that panels in other regions of the country might not fare well. Those guidelines had not been finalized by mid-2005. AIDS and gay groups are contending with this increased political pressure at a time when they have less money to do their jobs.

"We have a lot of work to do, but we desperately need resources," Dr. Barbara E. Warren, director of organizational development, planning and research at New York City's gay center, told *Metro Weekly*, a Washington, D.C., gay magazine, in 2005. "We have an opportunity here, but we also have a huge challenge."

Still, the community has responded to crystal with some resources beyond posters and town meetings. Those responses are effective. The growth in Crystal Meth Anonymous meetings, for instance, can be seen as evidence of the scope of the meth problem, but it is also evidence of a successful response to that problem. CMA is not alone.

A number of jurisdictions, including San Francisco, the states of California and New York, and New York City have dedicated hundreds of thousands of dollars to fund drug treatment efforts or research that specifically target meth users. Treatment not only gets the user off meth it can also reduce any unsafe sex that user might be engaging in.

A 2005 study of 162 gay and bisexual meth users in Los Angeles reported that treatment produced three-fold reductions in both drug use and high-risk sexual behavior among those men as well as reports of depression. These changes were "generally maintained over a yearling observation period."

In a press statement, Steven Shoptaw, the lead author on the study and a researcher at the Integrated Substance Abuse Programs at UCLA's Neuropsychiatric Institute, said, "The AIDS epidemic in the United States is integrally linked to drug use. Effective drug abuse treatments that produce lasting behavioral changes among addicts at risk of HIV are vital to prevention efforts."

This effect has been demonstrated before. A 1998 San Francisco study, which compared a harm reduction strategy to drug abstinence counseling, looked at two groups of gay men. All the men received counseling after abstaining from alcohol and drug use for thirty days. One group received counseling, the other received counseling plus a safe-sex intervention. Both groups reduced their unsafe sex by about half.

"Part of what they found was that substance abuse treatment was an effective HIV prevention strategy," said Joseph H. Neisen, executive director of New Leaf Services, a San Francisco mental health organization, in 1998.

The limits to drug treatment tend to be that there are not enough available treatment slots, the cost, and there are some specific issues that confront gay meth users, one being that, for a large number of gay meth users, sex and crystal are intertwined. One former user put it quite succinctly in a 2004 interview.

"Every time you get a hardon you're thinking about crystal," he said. Those gay users, fearing a hostile reaction, may not want to discuss their sex lives with heterosexuals.

"Most of the programs are putting them in with all the other amphetamine users," Dr. Dawn Harbatkin, medical director at the Callen-Lorde Community Health Center, a gay health clinic in New York City, said in 2004. "When you ask around that's the real deficiency with a lot of the groups. Gay men feel uncomfortable in the groups and they can't talk about their lives, their sex lives, and that's a big part of crystal use."

In an HMO era, the choices are also limited by money. Users who have private health insurance or who qualify for Medicaid, the government health insurance program for the poor or disabled, have the largest number of treatment options. Users who are uninsured have few.

"I've had many sad phone calls from friends who were trying to help friends," said Staley in 2004. "These people had no insurance and therefore they can't get quit. They're still on the drug. You just have to remove yourself completely from your surroundings when you're that addicted."

Private insurers may not want to pay for inpatient care and they may even limit the amount of outpatient care a user can receive. They may also differ with healthcare providers about what type of care is needed during the user's first days off the drug.

"Insurance providers claim that meth does not have a medically dangerous detox," said Marty Perry, executive director of the Pride Institute, which operates six drug treatment programs across the country. "Our belief is not that. We think that there are often medical dangers . . . Crystal is much more psychologically addictive, but the complicating thing is that there are a lot of physical things that happen when you are getting off it." These can include headaches, depression, sleep or skin problems, dehydration, and those who use a lot can experience paranoia to the point of being psychotic or delusional. Because crystal is not physically addictive, like heroin or nicotine, insurers may not pay to treat those problems.

While crystal has been around for decades, it has not received as much attention and research as other drugs, such as alcohol, cocaine, and heroin, have gotten over that time. Drugs to treat meth users may also become available. NIDA is developing medications to treat meth users. The agency established the Methamphetamine Clinical Trials Group in 2000 to conduct clinical trials on meth medications. Currently, it is reviewing two drugs.

While many media stories on meth present often present bleak futures for users and the communities they live in, the plain truth is that there are effective responses to meth and they are being used in the gay community and across the nation. The challenge for the broader community is apparent.

There are those who are declaring that methamphetamine is an "epidemic," a "scourge," or America's "number one" drug threat. What we have seen during earlier drug scares, such as with crack in the 1980s, is that such rhetoric by political and social leaders almost inevitably leads to standard and predictable responses.

The threat of the drug is often exaggerated and the hyperbole that accompanies a drug scare drives out the facts. As we saw with crack during the 1980s, certainly some, and perhaps a great deal, of the information on meth that has become part of the discourse on that drug is simply wrong.

There are no "meth babies," meth is not, as one *Rolling Stone* article put it, "instantly addictive," and users can stop using if they choose or if they get the appropriate help. People can use meth occasionally though one can certainly question the wisdom of that, given the potential health consequences, as well as the ethics of doing so, given that every meth purchase funds the misery that is associated with the drug.

Among gay men, the focus on crystal has led to a community that is no longer talking about the other drugs that also have deleterious health effects and can lead to unsafe sex. Despite the clear association these drugs have with unsafe sex, they have been pushed aside in our discussions about drug use though it must be said that the gay and AIDS groups that provide drug treatment services continue to aid users of these other drugs.

Meth has also taken attention away from the pressing issue of HIV among African-American and Latino gay and bisexual men who continue to experience unacceptably high rates of HIV incidence and prevalence. While the AIDS and gay groups that serve white, gay men have never been rich in resources, the groups that serve African-American and Latino gay and bisexual men are impoverished in comparison. An inordinate focus on crystal could do further harm to their budgets.

There are other parts of the broader community that have been forced out of the spotlight, or never allowed in, by the way in which gay men's health issues, most notably HIV and AIDS, have dominated the community discourse. Crystal may do that again.

In a 2005 *Metro Weekly* story, Sheila Healy, executive

director of the National Association of Lesbian, Gay, Bisexual, and Transgender Community Centers, noted that breast cancer, for instance, has taken a back seat.

"What's in this for women?" Healy said of crystal. "Women don't want to go on the back burner again over this issue."

Hysteria can also bring to bear the full law enforcement power of government and the cost of that is too often borne by drug users and not by the supposed "king pins" and "predators" who profit from the sale of illicit drugs. The often unjust results of that are already apparent in the gay community.

When three users—Peter K. Harris, Gary Kiss, and James Urinyi—receive disparate prison sentences simply because one was able to overcome his problem, a second conquered meth and cooperated with the government, while the third was unable to stop using crystal and received the harshest sentence of the three—that cannot be seen as a just result. No one should doubt that it is a good thing that Harris and Kiss were able to reduce their time in prison, but there is also no doubt that Urinyi was ultimately punished for his crime and for failing to stop using meth.

When Ronald "Sammy" Watkins and Kurt Douglas Guiterrez are given onerous prison sentences while Hans Reynoso, one of Watkins's drug suppliers, effectively walks away from prison because he entered into a cooperation agreement with the government who can reasonably endorse that result as fair, right or just? The two were punished as much for selling meth as for being unable to supply the federal government with useful information.

The price of joining the "war on drugs" is measured in many ways, but it certainly includes payment in freedoms lost, gay men imprisoned, and a community that is subject to intrusive government oversight.

These are not the only issues that confront the gay community when considering meth. Caleb Crain, author of the 1997 Lingua Franca story, wrote eight years ago, "For years, gays had managed to celebrate their successes in HIV prevention without confronting this stubborn remainder. But in late 1994, although the facts had not changed, the willingness of the gay community to talk about them had."

There certainly was talk in the 1990s, but there was not much more than talk. During the 1990s and into the twenty-first century, we saw a series of alleged epidemics—barebacking, bug chasing, men on the down low, and so on—that contributed nothing to gay men's lives or their health. Crystal may turn out to be just one more of these or it may draw our attention to that portion of the gay male community that cannot or will not take actions to keep themselves safe from HIV and other sexually transmitted diseases.

Those gay men who can take in information and alter their behavior to protect themselves and others will likely continue to do that though even they, as we have seen in recent years, are seeking help, but can we, finally, turn our attention to those men who are struggling?

This would not be easily done. It would require that the broader community demand that the local, state, and federal governments fund prevention, treatment, and other health efforts at levels that can effectively address these issues.

Such a demand would come after years of neglect of public health funding by government and when the priorities, certainly of our national government, are skewed toward aiding the richest in our nation and funding programs to counter terrorism, a phenomena that, in fact, poses no threat to the vast majority of Americans and a minor threat, if any at all, to just a few.

It would also require that those groups that serve gay men reject the fear-filled rhetoric and hysteria that characterizes much of the response to crystal in this country. Those groups must speak thoughtfully and reasonably to gay men about the problem that confronts us. They have to avail themselves of data and research to guide their efforts. They have to leave their offices and seek out the gay men they propose to assist. They have to do something that they have never done before—they have to lead. Then they have to do one more thing.

"The challenge for us is to really maintain our compassion within our own community," Warren said in *Metro Weekly*. "Not to let [crystal meth] vilify or demonize gay or bi men. Part of the crisis is the backlash. Some of the reasons that this behavior is so challenging is absolutely linked to the hostility and demonization of gay sexuality in our society. Using these drugs and these behaviors is a way to forget that . . . And twenty-plus years of dealing with an epidemic [that stifles sexuality] is very fatiguing."

FURTHER READING

Bayer, Ronald. *Private Acts, Social Consequences: AIDS and the Politics of Public Health*. New York. The Free Press, 1989.

Boykin, Keith. *Beyond the Down Low: Sex, Lies, and Denial in Black America*. New York. Carroll & Graf Publishers, 2005.

Feldman, Douglas A. and Thomas M. Johnson, eds. *The Social Dimensions of AIDS: Method and Theory*. New York. Praeger Publishers, 1986.

Garrett, Laurie. *Betrayal of Trust: The Collapse of Global Public Health*. New York. Hyperion, 2000.

Garrett, Laurie. *The Coming Plague: Newly Emerging Diseases in a World Out of Balance*. New York. Farrar, Straus and Giroux, 1994.

Inciardi, James A. and Karen McElrath, eds. *The American Drug Scene*. Los Angeles. Roxbury Publishing Company, 2004.

Rotello, Gabriel. *Sexual Ecology: AIDS and the Destiny of Gay Men*. New York, Dutton Books, 1997.

Shilts, Randy. *And the Band Played On: Politics, People and the AIDS Epidemic*. New York. St. Martin's Press, 1987.

Wolf, Michelle A. and Alfred P. Kielwasser, eds. *Gay People, Sex, and the Media*. New York. The Haworth Press, 1991.

$2^{\underline{00}}$ Gen 12/14 TA